Reiki

Reiki

THE ESSENTIAL GUIDE TO
THE ANCIENT HEALING ART

Chris and Penny Parkes
of The Reiki School

Vermilion
LONDON

11

This edition published in 2005 by Vermilion, an imprint of Ebury Publishing
A Random House Group company

First published 1998 by Vermilion

The Random House Group Limited Reg. No. 954009

Addresses for companies within the Random House Group can be found at
www.randomhouse.co.uk

A CIP catalogue record for this book is available from the British Library

Penguin Random House is committed to a sustainable future for
our business, our readers and our planet. This book is made from
Forest Stewardship Council® certified paper.

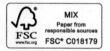

Printed and bound in Great Britain by Clays Ltd, St Ives plc

ISBN 9780091902490

To buy books by your favourite authors and register for offers visit
www.randomhouse.co.uk

Contents

PART TWO – REIKI TRAINING

PART THREE – HEALING WITH REIKI

Life is either a daring adventure,
or nothing.

HELEN KELLER

Preface

WE WERE DRAWN to Reiki shortly after the death of Chris's parents. We both felt we would have liked to do more to relieve their suffering during the last few months of their lives. We decided to take Reiki training both for our own self-healing and in the hope that we would be able to help others.

By the time we had taken First Degree Reiki, the cancer that was spreading through my mother's body had advanced rapidly. Her vibrant, colourful, positive character shone through her eyes, although her body had become very frail.

On one particular day, I noticed her parchment-like skin had become almost translucent as we wrapped her fragile frame in a warm blanket, put on some soft music and began to give her what had become a daily Reiki treatment. When we had finished, her face was animated and she began to describe an incredible vision she had experienced during the treatment. Prior to this time, my mother had always considered herself to be pragmatic and rational, drawn to the tangible rather than the ethereal. She was astonished to find herself describing, with some conviction, an experience that once she would have considered to be unreal.

Opposite the bed my mother lay on that day, there was a walk-in wardrobe room. The door was closed. She recounted that during the Reiki treatment she had become aware of a beautiful light streaming through the open door and seeing several brilliantly lit figures walking gently into her room. One of these figures was her late husband. She was almost overcome with emotion. The beings of light communicated to her that she need have no fear, that when the time came for her to leave her body, they would be there for her and an incredible experience awaited her. My mother told us she had never experienced such a vivid dream and described feeling filled with awe and tranquillity.

It was as if from that moment she was transformed. All fear and uncertainty had left her. She was filled with peace. Over the next few days, although she was weak, she put her affairs in order and had meaningful conversations with all close family members and certain friends.

My mother took the extraordinary step of preparing her large family for her impending death. Tissues were in short supply as this remarkable woman simply announced that it would all be over in approximately two weeks and that it was not the end, but a new beginning for us all. Her prediction was correct and her death was incredibly peaceful.

What a contrast this was to the final weeks in the lives of Chris's parents, who had passed away within ten months of each other a year or so previously. We had searched then for a better way to help relieve the discomfort, distress and fear they were clearly experiencing.

By the time my mother died, Chris and I knew that Reiki was something we wanted to do for the rest of our lives. This book is dedicated to the memory of my mother as well as my father, and to the memory of Chris's parents, who collectively taught us so much.

Penny Parkes

Introduction to the New Edition

MUCH HAS CHANGED SINCE THIS BOOK was published in 1998. Reiki has become well known and the perception of what was a largely unknown healing art has changed.

At the beginning of each course, I always ask people what has made them decide to take Reiki training and what they hope to gain from the course. In 1998, many of the students were therapists keen to learn a new skill in order to extend the range of treatments they offered.

Today, that has changed. People from all walks of life want to learn Reiki because they have seen how it has helped others and they are keen to have a powerful, enduring resource at their fingertips. People are in more need of healing than ever before. Busy, fragmented lives, without the certainties of times gone by, have led to fear-based responses, with increased numbers of people suffering from stress-related illnesses. Many feel their efforts simply don't secure the calm and fulfilment they are yearning for. With Reiki, they can find inner peace. After healing themselves, they can help others too. Little by little, Reiki has spread from person to person, from country to country, until it is now on every continent.

The aim of this book is to provide a practical, informative guide that contains everything a person would need to know about Reiki in order to gain the maximum benefit from its practice. Certain aspects have changed, such as the facts relating to Dr Usui's life. After Western practitioners became aware of the memorial on Dr

Usui's tombstone, we learned far more about the way in which he lived and how he came to discover Reiki. We believe readers of this book would enjoy hearing about his life and the way in which Reiki has evolved, but while we have updated this particular chapter and provided an overview, we have not dedicated a disproportionate amount of space to the history, as others have written books on this.

The focus of this book is to explain how Reiki works, what to expect from a treatment and how its practice can benefit you. In this updated edition, we also include empowering techniques, showing you how you can use Reiki to develop cast-iron self-confidence, endless energy and vibrant health, plus strategies to bring about positive change so Reiki can help you to live the life of your dreams.

In recent years, millions of Reiki enthusiasts throughout the world have developed many creative and wonderful ways of using Reiki to enhance their lives. I sincerely hope that the techniques shown here will help you create more happiness, peace and prosperity. Write and let us know of your successes, and who knows, they may be included in a future edition of this book.

In love, light and peace.

Chris Parkes

part one

REIKI —
UNIVERSAL
LIFE FORCE
ENERGY

CHAPTER ONE

Reiki – Energy For Life

THE WORD REIKI MEANS 'universal life force energy'. It refers to an ancient hands-on healing system founded by Dr Mikao Usui at the beginning of the twentieth century in Japan. The word itself is made up of two parts. The syllable *rei* (ray) describes the universal aspect of this energy, and *ki* (key) refers to the life force that flows through all living things. For thousands of years, numerous cultures, races and religions have been aware of the existence of a life force energy that corresponds to the meaning of *ki*. It is known as *chi* by the Chinese, *prana* by Hindus, *baraka* by Sufis, 'light' by Christians, *ruach* in Hebrew, and it is likely to have been known as *ka* by ancient Egyptians. In Japan, the energy is called *ki*, and it is from this word that Reiki is named.

Many ancient cultures have handed down knowledge of hands-on healing methods throughout history and have referred to the transference of a universal life force energy to promote well-being. Thousands of years ago, the ancient Tibetans had a profound understanding of the nature of matter and energy and used this awareness to heal their bodies, promote inner harmony and guide their spirits to an experience of wholeness and balance.

Later, such healing techniques were to emerge in India. Variations are also rooted in Chinese, Japanese, Greek, Roman, Egyptian, Native American and other ancient cultures. The secrets of such healing arts were carefully guarded and preserved by many of these cultures. Methods were handed down by word of mouth usually to priests or spiritual leaders and the knowledge was available to few in its entirety.

The art of Reiki might not have emerged at all had it not been for the persistence of Dr Usui, whose research led to the recovery of this ancient healing tradition in the early part of the twentieth century.

Energy fields

The scientific world has been aware for many years of what metaphysical and spiritual teachers have known for centuries. Our physical universe is not composed of any matter at all: its basic component is a kind of force, which could be called energy.

Seemingly solid items as perceived by our physical senses, such as a chair or a table, appear solid and separate from each other. On finer subatomic levels, however, such seemingly solid matter is made up of particles of energy. These particles vibrate at different speeds and it is this speed that holds the pattern of their physical form. Physicists describe particles not as isolated grains of matter but as interconnections in an inseparable cosmic web that interact with each other.

Physically we are all energy. Everything within and around us is made up of energy and we are all part of one great energy field. In *The Tao of Physics*, author Fritjof Capra says:

> *The exploration of the subatomic world in the 20th century has revealed the intrinsically dynamic nature of matter. It has shown that the constituents of atoms, the subatomic particles, are dynamic patterns, which do not exist as isolated entities, but as integral parts of an inseparable network of interactions. These interactions involve a ceaseless flow of energy manifesting itself as the exchange of particles; a dynamic interplay in which particles are created and destroyed without end in a continual variation of energy patterns. The particle interactions give rise to the stable structures. These build up*

the material world, which again do not remain static, but oscillate in rhythmic movements. The whole universe is thus engaged in endless motion and activity; in a continual cosmic 'dance of energy'.

Gary Zukav, in *The Dancing Wu Li Masters*, says: 'Quantum mechanics view subatomic particles as "tendencies to exist" or "tendencies to happen".' Such particles or patterns of energy have many different forms. Thoughts, for example, are a very fine, light form of energy, easily and quickly changed. Human tissue is also a light form of energy, influenced by many elements, and changes relatively quickly. A boulder is a denser form, slower to change and yet still affected by finer, lighter forms of energy such as water, for example. All forms of energy are interrelated and can affect one another.

Quantum physics suggests that the fabric of the universe is a form of energy and that all living beings are part of this field of energy. Gary Zukav writes:

> *. . . the philosophical implications of quantum mechanics is that all of the things in our universe (including us) that appear to exist independently are actually part of one all-encompassing organic pattern and that no parts of that pattern are really separate from it or from each other.*

As well as being composed of energy, we also have energy running through us. Many forms of medicine that originate in the East believe that it is this flow of energy that sustains life itself, and that this leaves the physical body at the time of death. This universal life force energy is said to pass through our systems via channels, which Orientals call the meridians of the body. In Chinese medicine, the aim of acupuncture is to stimulate the flow of energy through these pathways.

In optimum conditions, this vital energy flows unimpeded through our bodies and we experience good health and inner harmony. Conversely, during periods of stress or tension, it is reduced. This is when we usually experience pain, discomfort or distress. In the Chinese view, health is also affected by the interplay of two polar forces known as 'yin' and 'yang'. These represent cyclical patterns of motion and change. Yang represents the strong male, creative power and yin the female, receptive, maternal element. Disruption in the balance between these two forces is said to result in ill health. Balance between yin and yang is maintained by the continuous flow of energy through the body via the energetic grid or meridians. Should the flow of energy be restricted or blocked, well-being is affected.

Rather like the proprietary cleaners which disperse drain blockages in television advertisements, Reiki is said to dissolve such energy blocks by dissipating immobilised or slow-moving energy. The energy becomes drawn to the areas where the flow is slowed down or restricted and gently starts to break down the blockage. Gradually this life force energy is encouraged to flow freely again and help restore inner balance once more.

Particles of energy appear to be self-directing. Interestingly, Reiki energy does not generally need directing by the person giving the treatment. Gary Zukav describes how:

> The astounding discovery awaiting newcomers to physics is that the evidence gathered in the development of quantum mechanics indicates that subatomic 'particles' continuously appear to be making decisions! More than that, the decisions they make are based on decisions made elsewhere. Subatomic particles seem to know instantaneously what decisions are made elsewhere and elsewhere can be as far away as another galaxy! The key word is instantaneously! How can a subatomic particle over here know what decision another particle over there has made at the same time the particle over there makes it?

Reiki initiations

They key to Reiki, and one of the main differences between this and other healing modalities, is the initiation or attunement process, the catalyst for amplifying the life force energy.

WHAT IS AN ATTUNEMENT?

An attunement is a procedure in which the Reiki Master or teacher uses symbols and mantras to create a strengthened connection between the person and the universal life force energy. A series of attunements given by a suitably qualified Reiki Master is essential in order to become a channel for the energy.

Dr Usui, the founder, discovered how to use this energy as a beneficial healing treatment for others by employing the attunements to awaken and amplify the life force energy in anyone who has the desire to learn, so that they can become a recipient or a channel for the energy. He developed a system so simple that even a child could quickly learn to use it.

Reiki accelerates the healing process by supporting the body's natural ability to heal itself. As well as being a powerful tool for self-healing, it can be used to treat others. Additionally pets, plants and any living things can benefit too.

CHAPTER TWO

The Origins of Reiki

THE LATTER PART OF the 1800s was a transformational period in Japan's history and many changes were occurring throughout Japanese society. From 1639 up until 1854, the country had severed links with the outside world. Westerners were not allowed to enter and Japanese citizens forbidden to leave. When the Tokugawa shogunate fell in 1867, a new government was formed and the emperor declared the beginning of the Meiji era. Japan was no longer to be a closed society. The new emperor introduced Japan to modernisation and industrialisation after more than two centuries of isolation. Western culture poured into the country and was eagerly absorbed by citizens curious to know the benefits of scientific and technological advances. Those with knowledge of modern science were elevated to senior positions throughout Japanese society. Universities were founded, telegraph and railroads criss-crossed the land and a postal system was set up.

Into this environment of change and reform, Mikao Usui was born on 15 August 1865. His family was part of a privileged class. He was highly intelligent and well educated, graduating with a doctorate in literature. As an accomplished scholar, Dr Usui was widely read. He also spoke several languages and was knowledgeable on subjects as diverse as medicine, philosophy, psychology and theology. Whilst a practising Buddhist, he was also familiar with Taoism and Chinese scriptures. He is believed to have travelled extensively overseas, visiting both Europe and America as well as spending some time

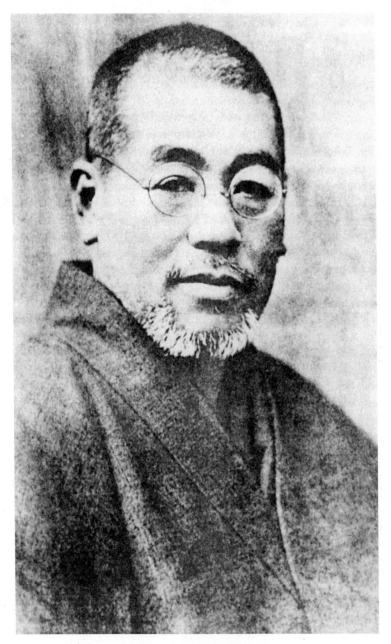

Dr Usui

studying in China. He was particularly interested in healing methods and studied both Japanese and Chinese techniques.

Dr Usui went into business whilst continuing the study of medicine and spirituality in his spare time. He later married and had two children, a son and a daughter. Through his studies, he became part of a Buddhist group whose centre was based at the foot of Mount Kurama Yama, near Kyoto. Dr Usui began to conduct his own extensive research into healing arts in the libraries and monasteries of Kyoto. Through his endeavours, he learned many techniques, and in time, he became a knowledgeable and respected teacher. He taught numerous ways to heal the illnesses that were prevalent in Japan. He also practised meditation and regularly went on retreat for solitude and spiritual advancement. On one of these retreats, he had an experience that changed the course of his life.

Dr Usui had decided to spend three weeks fasting and meditating on Mount Kurama. He collected twenty-one stones to act as his calendar, and would throw one away as each new day dawned.

For twenty days he meditated. Nothing out of the ordinary occurred. Then, just before dawn on the twenty-first day, Usui saw a flicker of light appear in the darkness. This light began to move quickly towards him. As it grew larger, Usui began to feel afraid. His immediate impulse was to retreat, but he decided not to move, even though he knew there was a risk. The light sped quickly towards him until it struck him on the centre of his forehead. He immediately slipped into a deep trance.

Usui later recalled that he thought at that moment he had died. He began to see strange symbols appearing before his eyes and became aware of information being imparted to him as each one came into view. When the vision faded, he awoke to find that it was now bright daylight and he was once again alone on the mountain.

He knew he had been given insight into a powerful healing method. Feeling energised and elated, he made his way down the mountain on his way back to Kyoto.

After taking some time to assimilate the knowledge he had received, Dr Usui went on to develop the system of healing we know today as Reiki. Initially he practised on family, friends and those

closest to him. He then began to offer treatments to those in need, and eventually, in 1921, opened a clinic in Tokyo and began to teach Reiki for the first time.

On 1 September 1923, an earthquake devastated Tokyo. More than 140,000 people lost their lives. A further 40,000 died as a result of a fire tornado which swept in from the sea. More than three million homes were destroyed and amenities such as the water and sewerage systems collapsed. It was estimated that over 50,000 people suffered serious injuries, and countless people were homeless. To assist, Usui and his students offered Reiki. The response was overwhelming. Many heard about the beneficial effects, and in early 1924 Usui built a larger clinic to handle the number of patients seeking treatment. Usui's reputation spread as a result of his humanitarian endeavours during the earthquake, and he was honoured by the Emperor of Japan. Many people wanted to learn Usui's healing method, and to meet demand he devised a more simplified form.

Over the next few years, he also began to train other teachers. One of these was a retired naval medical officer called Dr Chujiro Hayashi, who came to study with him in 1925. Hayashi had been with Dr Usui for about nine months, when on 9 March 1926, Usui unexpectedly suffered a stroke and died.

Dr Hayashi remained at Dr Usui's clinic for several years. He treated many people, taught Reiki and eventually left to found his own Reiki clinic in Tokyo. It was here that he modified the system, creating a number of degrees to represent the different levels of learning and developing a more complex set of hand positions suitable for clinical use.

In 1935 a Japanese–American woman from Hawaii came to the clinic. Mrs Hawayo Takata was a widow with two young children. She was suffering from depression plus a number of organic disorders. It was through Mrs Takata that Reiki was eventually to come to the West.

Mrs Takata was due to have surgery when she heard the voice of her late husband discouraging her from going through with the operation and urging her to find 'another way'. She wondered

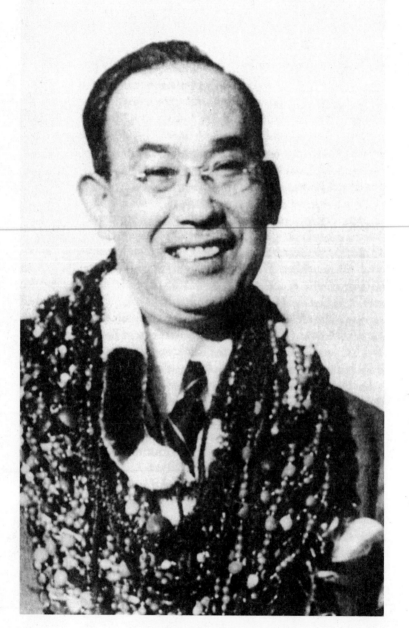

Dr Hayashi

initially if she was losing her mind, hearing voices. When the voice repeated itself for the third time, she decided to ask the chief surgeon if there *was* another way. He happened to have a family member who had been treated successfully at the Reiki clinic close to the hospital and suggested that treatment there would certainly be an alternative option. She subsequently decided against the operation.

Mrs Takata duly presented herself at Dr Hayashi's clinic for treatment. Initially very sceptical, she found herself becoming gradually more intrigued by this method of healing. She was treated by several practitioners at once and noticed how hot their hands became. At one stage, she was so convinced of trickery, she grabbed at the sleeve of a practitioner's kimono in an attempt to expose whatever was generating the intense heat she felt. She found nothing, and after being reassured by Dr Hayashi, she relaxed. After receiving treatments for several months, much to her own astonishment, Mrs Takata was healed.

Understandably impressed, Mrs Takata was keen to learn Reiki and bring it back to Hawaii. In the male-dominated Japanese society of that era, she met with considerable opposition, but eventually persuaded Dr Hayashi, who took her on as his apprentice. She lived with his family, learning and practising Reiki, for over a year, and was eventually initiated into First and Second Degree, later returning to Hawaii, where she began to practise. In 1938, Dr Hayashi initiated Mrs Takata as a Reiki Master in Hawaii, enabling her to teach and attune others to Reiki.

Towards 1940, Dr Hayashi knew that it was highly likely that Japan would enter the war, and as a former naval officer, he was expecting to be called up for military service. Having become a dedicated Reiki practitioner, however, he knew it would be impossible for him to serve even as a medical officer, as he no longer practised conventional medicine. In addition, because of his journeys to Hawaii, he also knew he was suspected of being a spy. Faced with an impossible choice between going to war or being imprisoned and executed, Dr Hayashi decided to take his own life. He died with dignity on 10 May 1940, in the company of his wife, as well as Mrs Takata and some of his students. He had passed on

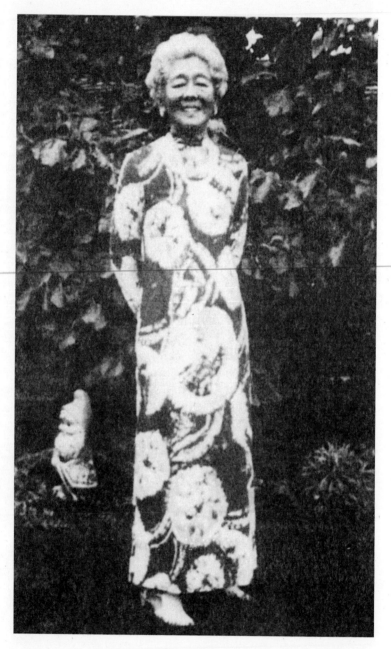

Mrs Takata

his knowledge to a number of his students in addition to Mrs Takata, who is believed to have been the last Master he taught.

Mrs Takata continued to practise Reiki in Hawaii for another forty years, though it was not until the 1970s that she began to train others as teachers. She died on 11 December 1980, having enabled more than twenty others to become Reiki Masters. Through these Masters, and others that have followed, Reiki spread to Europe and many other countries of the world. Their teachings are largely based on what was passed on by Mrs Takata. The popularity of Reiki has grown beyond anything Dr Usui could possibly have envisaged, and today people of all ages, cultures and backgrounds practise it on every continent.

CHAPTER THREE

How Reiki Differs from Other Therapies

ONE OF THE WAYS IN which Reiki differs from other healing methods is in the attunement of initiation process. Attunements or initiations are specific procedures (based on symbols and various techniques) carried out by Reiki Masters. They increase the individual's capacity for a greater amount of universal life force energy to pass through them. This source of energy is external and limitless. It benefits the healer's energetic system as well as the person receiving the treatment.

Another notable difference lies in the simplicity of Reiki. First Degree training is taught and learned in just a couple of days, though practice is later required. Reiki is easy both to learn and to apply.

Reiki symbols

The Usui System of Reiki differs from other healing arts in its use of symbols. Amongst other procedures, Reiki Masters use both symbols and sacred words during attunements to create the connection between the individual and the source of life force energy.

Treating yourself and others

Another difference is the way that Reiki can be used for self-treatment. The majority of people who decide to take Reiki First Degree training do so because of the advantages of being able to treat themselves. As a self-treatment, Reiki is simple and powerfully effective. Self-treatment can be administered anywhere at any time, quite inconspicuously. For example, it is easy to simply place your hands on your stomach whilst sitting on a bus or a train without drawing attention to yourself. Reiki is also an excellent way to minimise the effects of jet lag. There is usually plenty of opportunity on board to give yourself Reiki during the flight without anyone particularly noticing.

It is an invaluable tool for restoring depleted energy levels after a busy working day and can be used also to prevent illness developing. At the onset of a cold, a Reiki treatment can strengthen the immune system so that after a good night's sleep, the symptoms have vanished. Reiki is also effective as an emergency treatment for pain relief or to calm you down before an important event.

Treatment is given as a hands-on healing session that can last for over an hour. Usually the person lies down, fully clothed, facing upwards in a comfortable position on a treatment couch or any long flat surface (a bed or even a covered kitchen table will do). If it is a cool day, it may be appropriate to place a light blanket over the person receiving the treatment. It may enhance relaxation to play gentle background music. Some practitioners choose to place a few drops of essential oil of lavender (or another oil if preferred) in some water on a burner. However, these things are not essential.

Starting at the receiver's head, the practitioner then places their hands in a variety of positions on or above the body, each time for several minutes or more, while working slowly down the body. The person is then asked to turn over and the back is treated.

The energy soon starts to flow and treatment is usually deeply relaxing. Quite often the person being treated drifts into a light sleep. Each Reiki session is different, and experiences vary considerably.

EFFECTS OF REIKI TREATMENT

Reiki affects everyone in a different way. Experiences are determined by the needs of the person at the time. Usually a deep sense of peace and relaxation pervades.

During a treatment, heat or even a cool sensation is felt. Other responses include a fine vibration (even though the practitioner's hands are quite still throughout the treatment) or a nurturing feeling of being cocooned in a fine gossamer wave of energy. Sessions can sometimes provide much-needed inspiration, when new ideas unexpectedly spring to mind during or following a treatment. Some people find they want to take up a new interest or start a business venture.

Buried emotions can also surface during treatment. Repressed anger or fear may be experienced. Tears may even be shed. Too often we suppress aspects of our lives we are uncomfortable with, so that after some time they are no longer even in our conscious awareness. Once we are reminded, it can be a wonderful opportunity to recognise and deal with them, however difficult this may seem. Reiki has often been described as a catalyst to help develop conscious awareness. A symptom can simply be a message to help us to look within. Too often it is this non-consciousness which makes us ill. Reiki heightens awareness, and spontaneous emotional releases are not uncommon during treatments.

Many recipients fall asleep for the entire treatment and have no particular conscious awareness at all. This does not affect the outcome of the treatment. Reiki balances the system, and healing at a subconscious level occurs. Deep states of relaxation are experienced, with the person feeling refreshed as if they have slept for a long period. This is often accompanied by feelings of tranquillity and well-being. Very active individuals may find they wish to sleep more following treatment, and those who lack energy can feel energised.

Occasionally, it is possible to become aware of strong visual images during treatment, and even find the solution to a problem. Symptoms may diminish or disappear completely during treatment.

On rare occasions, slight brief discomfort may be experienced, as accumulated toxins are released. A pressured lifestyle combined with poor-quality food and not enough sleep, fresh air or relaxation can cause the body's elimination system to become sluggish. The

body may become used to a high level of toxins accumulating and being only partially released. Reiki treatments purify the system by speeding up the elimination of the body's waste products.

It is recommended that a large glass of water is drunk immediately after treatments and clients are advised to increase their overall intake of water or liquid to assist this toxic release. Reiki treatments can sometimes result in additional bowel and bladder movement and even increased mucus secretion or watering of the eyes. These are further symptoms of detoxification and indicate a natural cleansing mechanism at work.

The effects of Reiki are varied and unpredictable as this holistic treatment works on a number of levels, restoring wholeness and balance. A more in-depth appraisal of what might be experienced giving or receiving a Reiki treatment is covered in Chapter Ten.

Reiki for your pets

Reiki has proven to be an effective way of treating domestic pets of all kinds, as well as larger animals such as horses. Practitioners who work with animals on a regular basis tell us that they have been able to cut down on their vets' bills. The positive response of pets to Reiki is some proof of the astonishing effectiveness of this healing art, as animals are unable to respond to beliefs or psychology.

Generally, animals appear to enjoy receiving Reiki just as humans do, and quickly become calm when being treated. If it is not appropriate to treat a pet hands-on, then absent healing can be used to great effect. Animals instinctively know how much they need and often become restless once they have drawn an adequate measure of energy. Of course, we cannot know what they are experiencing, though usually they grow quieter whilst receiving the energy and become deeply relaxed just as humans do.

General principles of treatment would be to place your hands where pain is likely to be experienced by the animal and to allow your hands to remain there for a few moments. Then gauge the response, and if the animal is still relaxed, treat a few other body positions systematically.

When treating pets, it is a good idea initially to place your hands where the animal usually likes to be stroked. With the exception of cats, behind the ears is usually a good place to start. Cats can become restless quickly in this position. Alternatively, start by placing one hand on the head and one on the throat. Subsequently, go on to other areas on the body, just as you would with a human. Often, an animal will turn and adjust its position in such a way as to present the area that needs treating.

Hamsters, gerbils and other small animals can be treated by holding them in one cupped hand whilst placing the other hand slightly above them. Fish can be treated by placing hands directly on the aquarium and allowing fifteen or even twenty minutes for the energy to flow.

Horses respond well to Reiki and we have heard of horse breeders using it extensively. It has been particularly effective in accelerating relief from colic.

Family pets may exhibit indirect responses to Reiki too. Following our workshops, we are often told by participants that their pets run into the room at the beginning of a Reiki treatment. They usually make themselves comfortable on or under the table or couch and remain there until the treatment has been concluded. Pets often react in uncharacteristic ways after their owners have been attuned and take a short time to adjust to the changes. Passive pets have been known to suddenly charge round and round a room and then promptly settle themselves into the lap of their owner, where they remain for an unusually long time. Pets which are usually reserved often become much friendlier and more spontaneous.

Reiki for plants, shrubs and trees

Much has been written about the secret life of plants, and scientific tests have shown how they react to our emotions. Plant life is said to respond to love and care on an energetic level, and it would be difficult to dispute the therapeutic benefit of time spent gardening. Knowing this, it would not be hard to appreciate that plants, trees and shrubs can benefit from Reiki, just as humans and animals do. It could even be said that there is an exchange of energy as plants, in a subtle way, radiate back life-affirming properties.

To treat a houseplant, place your hands on either side of the base of the plant pot. After a moment you will feel the energy start to flow. After a few minutes the feeling will diminish, indicating that the plant has drawn enough. We have seen many ailing plants revive after a Reiki session. Houseplants enjoy being sprayed regularly with water. Keeping the leaves clean helps them to stay healthy and strong. Garden shrubs too benefit from Reiki. Trees can also be treated, either directly, by placing your hands on the bark, or indirectly, by sending Reiki using the absent healing technique taught at Second Degree level. Energy can be sent to a whole garden or park to help the trees and shrubs which have become weakened following stormy weather conditions, flooding or high winds.

There are only two ways to live your life. One is as though nothing is a miracle. The other is as if everything is.

ALBERT EINSTEIN

CHAPTER FOUR

Healing Yourself

I happen to believe that we make our own destiny. We have to do the best with what God gave us.

MAMA, FROM *FORREST GUMP*

Discovering your true purpose

As well as being a healing art, Reiki is also a path for personal development. As human beings, we all have a basic desire to contribute positively to the world and make a difference to fellow beings, as well as to improve and enjoy life as much as possible.

We acknowledge that each of us has a significant contribution to make, and in our hearts we are aware that we also have a higher purpose, even though it may not be apparent to us at a conscious level. The stresses and strains of life often distance us from the path that could lead to the fulfilment of our true destiny and may cause inner conflict, distress and possibly ill health. As well as enhancing physical well-being, Reiki usually increases mental clarity, restores emotional balance and deepens our spiritual connection. Intuition develops. We become more aware and in tune with our higher purpose. The subsequent decisions and choices that we make bring us back on course.

The adjustments might only be subtle and inconsequential initially. In time, however, these alterations amount to substantial changes. It may be that by simplifying our lives and organising ourselves better, we are able to work one hour less each day. This could enable us to be home early to spend more time with the family or enjoy the sunset. One day, after witnessing a marvellous spectacle of nature, we might be further inspired to take up a new hobby, from which eventually a rewarding career is launched. A subtle change can sometimes shift regular patterns of living in such a way as to allow you to enjoy life more fully and more closely aligned with your higher purpose.

Harnessing the power within

Inner transformation can occur on a number of levels. Our experience of life is often restricted by the limitations of our own beliefs. Our thought processes may alter completely, as self-awareness grows.

Our thoughts powerfully influence our experience of life. Some of these are positive and uplifting. Others are negative and limiting. For example, two people might choose to visit a large city. One person might believe that cities are terrible, unsafe places where cars are stolen, people are overcharged and noise levels are unacceptably high. The other might believe that cities are exciting, thrilling places to visit, where it is possible to enjoy magnificent cultural attractions, sophisticated shops and stimulating people. Both would clearly have different experiences in that city, even from the same vantage point; one noticing only traffic, litter and pollution and the other seeing the parks, the architecture and the creative window displays.

Negative thoughts can ultimately prevent us from achieving our full potential. Increased clarity through Reiki can help us to become aware of and even eliminate negative beliefs, allowing us to gain a deeper understanding of others and ourselves.

This awareness can develop understanding of the relationship between negative thoughts and physical problems. Many psychotherapists agree that strong emotions are frequently internalised within the body. Often at the point in therapy when the clients release limiting beliefs about themselves, their aches and pains sponta- neously disappear. Similarly deep-tissue body-workers, such as those who practise holistic massage, find that therapy releases strong emotions, and it is not unusual to find treatments provoking a healing crisis as repressed feelings surface. When this happens, healing begins.

Reiki can help you to release physical tension and mental stress, as well as generating feelings of confidence and optimism. This encourages a far more positive outlook in times of stress. It also helps you to face uncertainty and make decisions from a more balanced perspective. The process is cumulative, and continues each time a treatment is received. In this gentle but powerful way, Reiki supports you on your journey of self-healing and helps you to harness your inner power.

part two

REIKI
TRAINING

CHAPTER FIVE

First Degree

THERE ARE FOUR LEVELS of energy in the Usui System of Reiki. The first is the introductory level, or Reiki First Degree as it is generally known. The next is Reiki Second Degree. The third is called Master Practitioner or Advanced and the final level is the Master Teacher level.

First Degree Reiki training is made up of four sessions, usually with one attunement per session. These sessions often take place over a two-day period, such as a weekend, or alternatively can be held over four evenings. Each Reiki Master will bring his or her own variations to this basic structure. Mrs Takata, who brought the Usui System of Reiki to the West, taught the four sessions over four consecutive days or evenings. Whilst the scheduling today varies enormously, the format of the training remains virtually the same as it was when Mrs Takata taught Reiki.

The courses usually comprise four attunements (although this can vary depending on the teacher), the telling of the Reiki story, the five ethical principles, the hand positions, and instructions for self-treatment, the treatment of others and the treatment of injury. Energy perception is usually also taught, and there is often time to practise what has been learned.

The remaining components of the workshop rely on the personality, ability and interests of the particular Reiki Master. There may even be variations between the classes any one Reiki Master holds, depending on the particular group energy of the participants.

Courses do vary. In our experience it is preferable for the training to be held over a two-day period, so there is adequate time to integrate the experience. Some teach Second Degree training straight after the First Degree course. In our opinion, this has never been a good idea, as a period of growth is triggered following the First Degree attunements and it is important to allow some time to process the changes.

Some Reiki Masters recommend participants have no heavy meals, alcoholic drinks, or drugs (with the exception of prescribed medication) over the three-day period prior to and following training. Smaller classes are preferable, with approximately twelve to fifteen participants per class (although larger classes are acceptable if there is more than one Reiki Master present). It is important that each participant is able to receive personal attention from a Reiki Master.

A typical format for the first day would include the first two attunements. Additionally, the history of Reiki, including the five ethical principles, is covered, along with full details of how to give yourself a self-treatment, instructions for the twenty-one-day cleansing period, and lots of practice (see Chapter Ten – Treating yourself: the twelve basic positions).

We often advise participants to start keeping a journal to observe the changes that occur over this period and beyond. As well as being attuned on the first day, students may also become acquainted with the universal principles of energy flow, so they are able to direct it to where it is required in their lives.

On the second day, two further attunements usually take place. There may also be tools and techniques for using Reiki not only for healing, but also as a path for personal and spiritual growth. Participants are taught how to give a Reiki treatment to others. Details of how to develop intuitive and kinaesthetic sensitivity, as well as practical knowledge for setting up a treatment room, may be given. In addition, information such as how to use Reiki to help people through a difficult period in their lives, and how to recognise and support them through a healing crisis, might be included. This is usually followed by a practical one-to-one session when all participants give and receive a full Reiki treatment. There should be plenty of time for questions and answers throughout the training, with ample opportunity for sharing any experiences.

Reiki is an oral tradition and there is usually no need to take notes, although some may prefer to.

By the end of the training, most people have had a very positive experience and leave feeling light-hearted, relaxed and loving. Some even have deeply moving spiritual experiences during the attunements, and others feel extremely relaxed, though not aware of any significant occurrence.

We are often asked why Reiki training is divided into three stages. This is because in Dr Usui's day, students would travel with him, learning and practising Reiki, until eventually they too were ready to teach. This is not a practical option today, and in modern times it is simply easier to divide the attunements into degrees to allow the necessary time to assimilate the various levels of energy amplification.

The attunement is a very special time during which the student may become conscious of an inner world unfolding. We advise each person to close his or her eyes and go within, as it is best not to be distracted by the external physical world.

Bringing change into your life

Following the attunements, a number of changes may occur. The vibratory rate of each individual is raised, and although the effects are subtle, the overall difference may bring considerable changes into the lives of participants. These might include:

- Becoming more intuitively aware and generally more sensitive to energies. This continues to develop, especially when the energy is being channelled either during a self-treatment or when treating others.
- Becoming more responsive and loving due to increased awareness of your feelings and emotions. Subsequently you can become more sensitive to your own needs, as well as to the needs of others.

- Increased awareness and clarity leading to a shift in perception. The mind becomes clearer and often our decision-making process is sharpened.

Other changes that may be noticed are:

- Changes in diet. Often showing a preference for food that carries a finer, lighter vibration. Some people decide to change their diet to increase the amount of fresh produce. Manufactured foods may lose some of their appeal.
- Overcoming addictions. Many people spontaneously stop smoking after taking Reiki training. Some people no longer feel the need for a 'smoke screen' between themselves and the world.
- Improved focus, memory and concentration. Many students have reported improvement to their concentration span. Practitioners say their meditation deepens following their attunements.
- Some notice a different response from family members, friends, colleagues, pets, etc. Some observe stray animals coming up to them in the park and strangers in the supermarket engaging them in conversation.
- New interests emerge. Many people unexpectedly decide to take up new hobbies, discover talents they were unaware of, or unexpectedly change their jobs, or even their professions.

The five ethical principles

Dr Usui adopted these five ethical principles in his teachings, as he realised the importance of a person's participation in his or her own healing process. A person needed to ask for help and be active in bringing change into his or her life. He appreciated that healing the spirit was paramount and that this required commitment and a degree of personal responsibility to be effective. These guidelines were developed to help people to grow and change and are as relevant today as they were during Dr Usui's lifetime.

JUST FOR TODAY, DO NOT WORRY

This reminds people that there is a divine purpose to everything, and that without awareness of this, further limitations may be created. Taoist sages declare that 'any event in itself is neither good nor bad, it simply is'. Energy used for worrying is in essence wasted, as it brings no change to a situation. Dr Usui used this principle to remind people of the importance of trust. We live in a responsive universe, and as long as we are clear as to what we want, our needs will be met. Sometimes it is important to simply trust that things will work out for the best in the end. What is beyond our control cannot be changed, and squandering copious amounts of our energy on worrying may only serve to diminish our vitality and cloud our perception.

JUST FOR TODAY, DO NOT ANGER

When a situation does not live up to our expectations, we can become angry. Anger is a destructive emotion when expressed inappropriately. Anger can also be a powerful motivator for change, provided you are able to become consciously aware of your reactions and take charge of your emotions. It would be inappropriate to feel guilt if anger arises. Anger creates disharmony within the body. Dr Usui was not asking people to deny their feelings. Instead he was asking them to respond with love.

EARN YOUR LIVING HONESTLY

A sage was once asked to explain how it was possible to gauge how prosperous someone was. He thought for a moment and replied that the measure of how prosperous a person was depended upon the amount of peace they could carry in their heart. When a person earns their living honestly, they are not only being honest with others, they are being honest with themselves. They trust in their own abilities to create the abundance they need, to provide for themselves and their families. Such persons would indeed carry more peace in their hearts and would be immeasurably well off. Dr Usui, in using this principle, was aware that dishonesty was a heavy burden to carry. He believed that people could align themselves more fully with their life's purpose and their creativity if they were to earn their living honestly.

SHOW GRATITUDE TO EVERY LIVING THING

Gratitude allows us to open up to the fruits of the universe and create a conscious awareness that magnetically attracts abundance and repels lack. There is a well-known universal principle that 'like attracts like'. Dr Usui knew that feeling and showing gratitude could enable people to bring success, prosperity and happiness into their lives.

HONOUR YOUR PARENTS, TEACHERS AND ELDERS

This principle of showing love and respect for our parents, teachers and elders may well be extended to every living thing. All living things are interdependent. Man's inhumanities to his fellow man and to the environment have caused many humanitarian and ecological problems. In order for the planet as a whole to survive, mankind must change. Dr Usui appreciated that our growth and indeed our survival depended on loving actions, self-respect, and respect for one another and all living things. The first place to start is with our loved ones and those close to us; not of course, forgetting ourselves in that important process. Taking positive action and responding sensitively, with warmth and compassion, towards parents, teachers, elders and subsequently everyone you encounter from now on will go some way towards reducing the suffering in the world around us.

The importance of an energy exchange

To live in balance and harmony, it is helpful to feel comfortable with the concept of giving and receiving, which is the essence of an exchange of energy. The exchange of energy does not always have to be in the form of money; it can be any form of exchange that is acceptable. Amongst close family members and friends, exchanges of energy are frequent anyway and specific requests are usually unnecessary.

To reduce the burden of obligation, an exchange of energy is an important part of the healing process. It is far better to treat people who are keen and willing to transform themselves, than those not interested or prepared to receive.

For Reiki treatments, it is usually recommended that the charge is comparable to the cost of a body massage in your areas. Most practitioners offer concessions to those unable to afford a treatment. Similarly, Reiki Masters usually offer reduced fees to students who wish to learn and are unable to afford the full tuition cost.

Giving a Reiki treatment

Each of the hand positions has a specific significance and can provoke different reactions from both the healer and the person being treated. The person giving the treatment receives the energy running through their system and benefits from the treatment too. The energy heightens perception and sensitivities and is a special time for both healer and recipient. There are many more hand positions and guidelines than the basic ones described here which are often taught at First Degree level. When giving first aid, it is usual to place hands directly on to the area that needs treating. There are a number of books with specific hand positions for a variety of illnesses and conditions, including our book *15-Minute Reiki*, which deals with many common ailments and specific hand positions to treat them. Some may be discovered intuitively whilst giving a treatment. Flexibility is important, and it is as well to remember that Mrs Takata taught Reiki as an intuitive art, not as a rigid system.

How to determine the most appropriate hand positions

Except for shock or accident, give Reiki to the entire body whenever possible, as the body is a complete unit and should be treated as a whole. If you have a short space of time for treatment and can only do a limited number of hand positions, it is possible to determine where the optimum positions are by:

- Directly treating the area of discomfort.
- Using intuitive abilities to tune in and to discern which areas most need the energy.
- If you are familiar with acupuncture meridian points, giving Reiki over the area that corresponds to the symptom.
- If you are familiar with reflexology points in hands and feet, giving Reiki to the corresponding area.
- Observing where the person receiving the treatment places their hands instinctively. This is often where it is most needed.

Hand positions for giving a full treatment

FIRST POSITION

This first position is over the eyes, forehead and cheeks. The heel of the hand is the only part of the hand that should be in contact with the person, resting on their forehead. This position affects the pituitary and pineal glands as well as the eyes, sinuses, nose, teeth and jaws. It also helps to reduce stress and aid the processes of thought and concentration. It is the natural position used to treat a headache and for colds of the nasal and frontal sinuses. It also assists in awakening the third eye. Many cultures have depicted the third eye as the energy centre from where our perceptive and intuitive abilities originate. For further details see page 79.

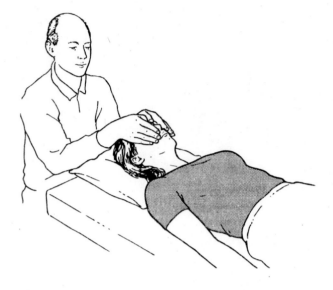

SECOND POSITION

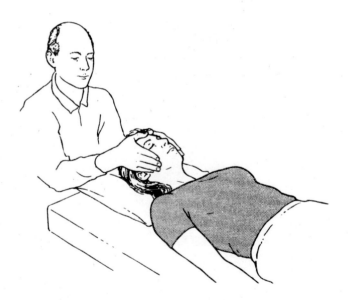

Move the palms of the hands to the temples with thumbs over the third eye. This affects the brain and the eye muscles. It is also good for colds, headaches and seizures, as well as the pituitary and pineal glands. It assists with shock and motion sickness, and helps relieve worry, hysteria, stress and depression. This position enhances dream and past life recall. It creates calmness and improves memory retention, productivity and creativity.

THIRD POSITION

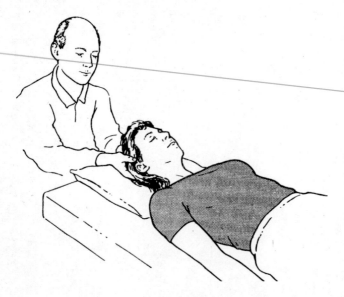

Moving your hands to the back of the head and base of the skull affects weight and vision. It assists with speech and controls the nervous system for the entire body. It also helps to relieve stress and promotes relaxation. It relieves pain and nausea and enhances dream and past life recall. At a mental level it calms thoughts and helps relieve depression.

FOURTH POSITION

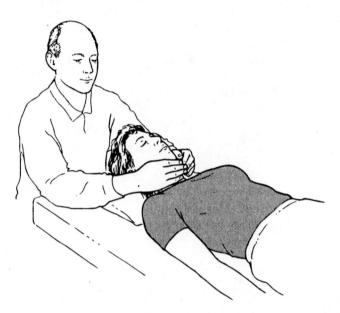

Place your hands over the throat and along the jawline. This position assists with strokes, tonsils, throat, larynx, thyroid and parathyroid and helps in balancing blood pressure. It improves lymphatic drainage and brings calmness and clarity of thought. It also helps the vocal cords, and conditions like anorexia, metabolic diseases and weight problems. In addition, it helps to bring confidence and joy. It relieves anger, hostility and resentment. It is important not to touch the neck when treating, as this would cause discomfort and concern to the person being treated.

FIFTH POSITION

This position is over the heart and treats the heart, lungs and thymus, which in turn affect the immune system and circulation. At an emotional level, this facilitates the release of stress and assists in enhancing the capacity to give and receive love. At a

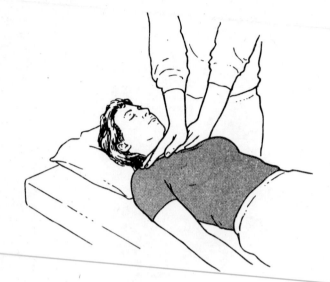

mental level, it helps the process of relieving depression and contributes towards restoring balance and harmony.

SIXTH POSITION

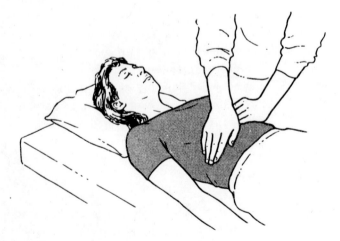

This position is just below the chest, still on the rib cage and over the solar plexus area. It affects the liver, stomach, spleen, gall bladder and digestion. It also helps to bring relaxation and to release fears and stress. At a mental level, it helps bring about inner balance.

SEVENTH POSITION

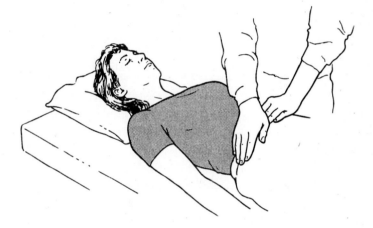

The seventh position is over the abdomen area and affects the liver, pancreas, gall bladder and transverse colon. This area is the centre wherein angry thoughts and words are held, creating feelings of bitterness, blame and frustration. When energy is brought to this area, it assists in releasing negative thoughts. This is a very calming position.

EIGHTH POSITION

This position is over the pelvic area and affects lymphatic drainage and the release of toxins. In addition, it brings energy to the large and small intestines and the bladder. It assists with issues of constipation and diarrhoea and affects the ovaries, uterus and prostate. This centre also

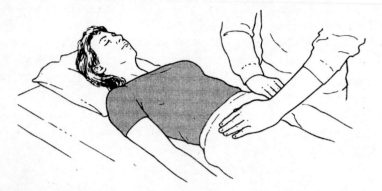

relates to feelings of security and pleasure. It is the area of creativity and elimination, allowing the release of unneeded, outdated ideas and substances.

KNEES AND FEET POSITION

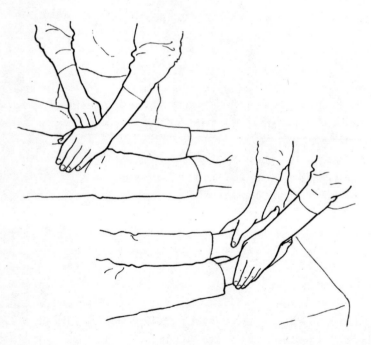

Take the energy down the legs to the knees. The knees often store repressed emotions and even anger. Treating the knees for a moment or two is often soothing and both hands may feel as if they really want to stay longer, which is a sign that this area is benefiting from the energy. Then move on down to the feet and place the hands around the ankles for a while, working towards the toes. After this point, the person is asked to turn over. Even if they have been asleep, it is amazing how they usually wake up briefly to turn over and then drift straight back to sleep.

NINTH POSITION

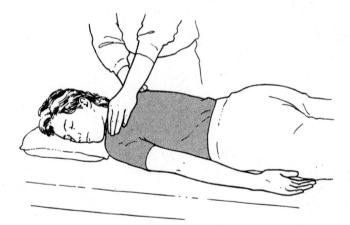

This position is at the top of the shoulders and affects the heart as well as the shoulders and neck. It facilitates the release of stress and burdens and brings peace and harmony. Tension is often stored in this area. It can give rise to the feeling of 'carrying the weight of the world on the shoulders'.

TENTH POSITION

This position is over the shoulder blades and at a physical level affects the heart and the lungs. At an emotional level, it enhances the ability to love and be loved, as well as facilitating the release of stress. At a mental level, this position brings peace and harmony.

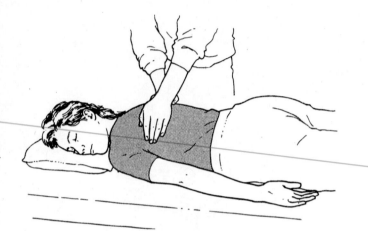

ELEVENTH POSITION

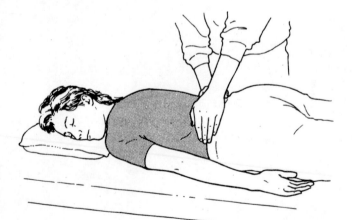

The eleventh position is over the lower back. This affects the gall bladder, pancreas, transverse colon, adrenal glands, kidneys and lower back. It assists in releasing self-criticism, anxiety and negativity. It allows feelings of harmony and joy to surface.

TWELFTH POSITION

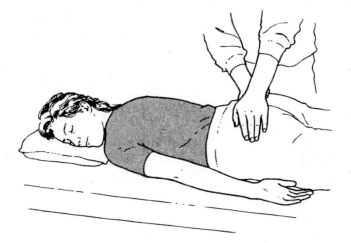

This position is over the tailbone and affects the large and small intestines, bladder, uterus, ovaries, prostate and coccyx. This area is also associated with creativity and releasing. Here the releasing of old thoughts and feelings makes room for new innovative, creative expressions to emerge.

CONCLUDING THE TREATMENT

After the twelfth position, we recommend the energy be taken briefly down to treat the soles of the feet, benefiting the reflex zones. As many people will be driving after the session, or certainly will need to be alert, it is helpful to then take the energy back up to the head.

To do this, place both hands in line pointing up the spine, about a hand width apart, one hand on the base of the spine and the other between the shoulder blades. Briefly smooth the energy out across the back of the spine, working from both sides of the top of the spine in even sweeping motions outwards, all the way to the back of the hips. This is a different movement and will help to bring the person round and let them know the treatment is coming to an end. Finally, 'sweep the aura free' of any accumulated debris by using sweeping movements from the head to the toes in the auric field slightly above the body. We usually recommend disposing of this debris by visualising it floating away. The aura is the subtle energetic field surrounding and penetrating the body. It is an energetic composition of the body's structure and functions, as well as containing a person's thoughts, feelings and awarenesses.

At this point, the person may be coming round a little and it would be appropriate to let them know that there is no hurry and that you are leaving them for a brief moment to give them some time to wake up. This is an appropriate time to wash your hands and bring back glasses of water for both yourself and your client.

Allow a little time for feedback from the person being treated and advise them to drink more water than they usually would over the next few days to assist any toxic release. For the same reason, it is also helpful to suggest that they take more showers and refrain from drinking alcohol over the next 24–48 hours.

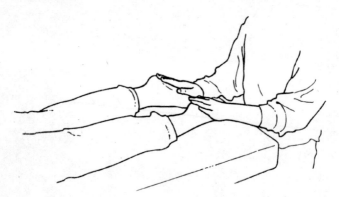

Developing your intuitive perception

A simple and powerful method for assessing the energetic requirements of each person is to use the hands to scan the body in order to receive impressions of energy imbalances. Initially, energy perception can be very subtle. It usually takes time, practice and focus to develop this awareness, though it can be surprising how quickly this ability grows.

SENSING ENERGY

To sense energy, rub the hands briskly together and hold them about three feet apart. Now bring the hands together, slowly, noticing when there is slight resistance. This very subtle, intangible resistance is the energy. Keep trying until you can get a sense of it.

When you are giving Reiki treatments, your hands become your inner eyes, trained to perceive the areas that need attention.

SCANNING THE BODY

When you are comfortable with the above exercise and have a sense of what energy feels like, use the hands to scan the body to pick up any impressions. You might want to practise on family and friends at first.

To scan the body, rub the hands briskly together and hold them over the person's head in the auric field. Move them up higher and then lower to try to get an impression how far the immediate energy field stretches. In a healthy person, this should be well above the body. Then move the hands slowly through the auric field from the person's head to their feet. Notice any differences in heat or variations in the depth of the energetic field, and any other impression that you are able to sense. This takes some practice. Don't worry if it doesn't happen immediately.

It is helpful to scan each person before their treatment, to assess which areas need to be concentrated upon. It is important to scan once and once only, as it can be disconcerting to the person lying on the treatment table to have you go up and down their body repeatedly, and may make them curious as to what you are doing and unnecessarily anxious about what you might be picking up.

Provided the person knows generally what to expect during a treatment, it is not even that important to explain that you are scanning their body and hoping to receive impressions. It could be of concern to someone that you are spending more time over their heart, for example, which might give them the idea that they are about to experience a heart attack. If you appear to be holding back on any impressions received, it may be feared that you are concealing vital information.

Having completed the body scan, go on to treat the body. Bear in mind any areas you feel are particularly important to concentrate on. Notice any particular sensations in the area that the person has requested you spend time on.

Guide to the meaning of impressions received

As each person gains experience, his or her sensitivity will develop. What was almost too subtle to recognise initially will become more obvious with practice. The next step is to interpret these subtle variations. We have compiled a list of typical energetic impressions that are common to most practitioners, and their general meanings in our experience.

VISUAL IMPRESSIONS

The practitioner can often receive visual impressions. It may or may not be appropriate to discuss them with the person. If you know them well enough, and feel they might be receptive, then tactfully communicate your observations. Otherwise, remain silent, as it may not be appropriate, helpful, or in the person's best interest to mention images that could be misunderstood and could cause someone to feel uneasy.

HEAT

This indicates that the energy is needed in this area and is being drawn (when the practitioner experiences a greater flow of energy through themselves to the individual). Strangely, sometimes the heat can be intense and it may even be necessary to break contact for a moment if the recipient is uncomfortable. This is unusual. One person was receiving Reiki for a headache. The practitioner's hands were placed on both sides of this person's head. He experienced warmth on the right-hand side of his head only and was curious to know why this should be. When asked where his headache was, he confirmed that it was in the area experiencing the heat, which was why he was drawing more of the energy in that area. Heat is often experienced when the energy is drawn to a symptom of a physical nature.

COOLNESS

This usually suggests an energetic block of some sort in the area, where there seems to be little energetic movement. Not much energy is being received and the corresponding chakra may be malfunctioning. (The sanskrit word chakra means wheel and refers to the various points on the body through which energy passes. For more details see Chapter Eleven.) Often, coolness experienced by the recipient can indicate blocks of an emotional or even a spiritual nature. There may also be repressed feelings. The exercise to clear energy blocks in Chapter Eleven may help. Deep inner work is often necessary to start the process of releasing. Treating the whole body will help to free up the energy in this area.

TINGLING

This sensation can indicate the presence of inflammation, or bruising. If there is no obvious cause of the inflammation, there may be suppressed anger. The knee and jaw often store a lot of emotion; there might also be anger trapped there. Reiki is effective in allowing deep-seated feelings and emotions to surface, after which the tingling sensation diminishes rapidly.

HANDS FEEL STRONGLY DRAWN TO AN AREA

This indicates an area in need of healing. Usually the energy is being freely drawn. Sometimes our hands unconsciously remain in a position for a long time. It will be as though your hands are stuck there for a while. This often happens naturally when more energy is required in a particular area. When the energy begins to ebb you will know it is time to move on to the next position.

HANDS FEEL REPELLED FROM AN AREA

This usually implies that there is an old deep-seated issue the person is reluctant to face. There is likely to be an energetic blockage in the area that is resisting the energy at all costs. This could be because of an earlier experience or event. It could even result from a past-life trauma. It is important to ascertain whether the client feels ready to deal with such deep-rooted blockages. If there is fear, then the person is not ready. If this is the case, it is probably best to leave this area alone for the time being and perhaps send absent healing to the person to help heal the cause.

DULL PAIN

This often implies there has been a physical problem in the past.

Perhaps there is scar tissue in this area, which has caused a build-up of energy. The body's immune system will naturally deal with such areas and Reiki will help accelerate that healing process.

SHARP PAIN

This may pinpoint an area where there is a build-up of energy that urgently needs releasing. Concentrating on this area will help to break it down and allow the free flow of energy once more. Whole body treatment is advised, rather than treating this area in isolation, although it may need more focus initially.

VIBRATION

This may indicate the chakra has been under- or over-functioning in this area and energy is being drawn through, to balance and repair it. Often the person may be unaware of the vibration. Alternatively, they may have felt a strong vibration, whilst your hands experienced no movement at all. The hands will not be moving in any event. It will be the way in which the energy is moving that is causing the vibration.

It may be confusing when the person's impressions do not coincide with your own, and this is because they are processing the experience differently. Their own observation will personalise their experience of the energy. The person receiving the treatment may experience the energy totally differently to the healer. That is quite usual. The above is a general guide only, and many people will interpret their impressions differently, in their own way.

Some practitioners find that inner abilities begin to emerge gradually as they progress through the various levels. This is a result of the strengthened connection to the energy and can be most helpful in determining areas of imbalance within a person. Developing intuitive abilities can be a useful by-product of Reiki practice, but guard against attaching too much importance to psychic 'messages'. This can lead to self-deception and a tendency to over-interpret everything. Suddenly a treatment becomes a psychic reading. Unless one has done a lot of inner work, there can be a tendency to operate out of one's projections, perceiving them to be real. We have seen many people deluded by their awakening abilities, believing them to be an end in themselves. Such sensitivity can be a useful diagnostic tool, but it is not much use having these abilities simply to impress others for the sake of it, or to boost one's ego into believing you have an infallible power. This is when self-deception can cloud the issue, rather than clarifying it. Some Reiki Masters attach too much importance to the development of 'psychic abilities' as an end in itself. It is helpful to remember that you are working with Reiki to help others, and ego-inflating displays of clairvoyant ability may not necessarily be beneficial to the recipient.

Reiki is taught differently in the East, where there is more focus on teaching sensitivity to the energy. This is because many Japanese techniques have their roots in traditional Eastern energy medicines, such as acupuncture, which seeks to treat health according to the flow of *ki* or *chi* energy through a person's system. In the West, techniques have been added on by individual Masters, often with some New Age influences, and Reiki has evolved slightly differently. Links have been made to spiritualism, with much emphasis on spirit guides. In essence, the Eastern and Western approaches are broadly similar. In practice, there are differences. First Degree courses should ideally contain at the very minimum:

Twelve hours of tuition
Four attunements
The hand positions
Treatment of self and others, with time to practise
The five ethical principles
Energy perception

CHAPTER SIX

Second Degree

THE SECOND DEGREE CLASS enables the participant to become a channel for a far greater amount of life force energy than at First Degree level. We recommend that you allow at least three months in between First and Second Degree in order to assimilate the energy. There is usually one initiation at Second Degree level. A further level of energy is activated at this level and a twenty-one-day cleanse is again recommended to enhance the integration of this energy.

Following initiation at Second Degree level, the energy flows through the system in greater quantities. When self-treating or treating others, just three minutes instead of five will suffice in each position as a general guide. There are circumstances which may dictate otherwise, such as in first aid applications. The energy at this level focuses particularly on emotional and mental healing of the individual, and is far more intensive. This level is particularly helpful for professional therapists who incorporate Reiki into their existing treatments and work to a time schedule.

We still recommend an hour when giving a full treatment to another person. A person's system will usually draw as much energy as is needed within three minutes in any one position. This also allows the practitioner to concentrate on the stressed areas without greatly extending the overall session time.

This course is usually divided into two or three sessions that can either be held over two days (a weekend, for example), or over three evenings. As in First Degree, the format varies with individual Reiki Masters. One session may include the attunement, another the three symbols, plus additional information relating to their use. The third session may focus entirely on the absent healing technique and the stronger form of mental and emotional healing. Usually the training is lively and exciting as the material contained at this level is fascinating, stimulating and thought-provoking.

Intuition and Second Degree

The third eye, if it has not been sufficiently stimulated at First Degree, will certainly be at Second Degree, increasing the perceptive abilities of participants. Some students at this level find they become able to perceive energy fields and auras. Clairvoyance or intuitive abilities may develop. As time goes on, it is often easier for a person who has taken this level to receive information at an intuitive level, as the Second Degree initiation works directly on the etheric body. The connection to the higher self is also strengthened by the attunement at this level.

To develop intuition, it is important to be able to differentiate between impulses and inspired intuition received from our higher selves. Intuitive thoughts and messages are often accompanied by feelings of peace and harmony. They can be strong or vivid, subtle or light impressions or thoughts that leave us in no doubt. They usually recur at least three times. Impulses and desires conversely can evoke a sense of urgency or anxiety, putting you under pressure. They often feel as though they must be carried out immediately. It is helpful to take a moment to distinguish between the two.

Reiki symbols

At this level, three symbols are taught, as well as the mantras that activate them. Each of the symbols is learned by heart and committed to memory. Afterwards instruction is given on how and when to use them. There have been many books written about symbols, describing them as the universal cosmic language.

Distant healing

This method allows a person to send healing to recipients who are not physically present. The approach uses symbols and a specific technique to connect with a person or any living thing and send energy to them as if they were in the same room. All that is needed to start the process of establishing an energetic bridge across which energy can be transmitted is their name and a picture, or perhaps simply bringing their image to mind.

This technique also offers the possibility of being able to send energy to numerous recipients simultaneously. Sometimes, once the connection has been established, it is possible to receive a response as well. We have been told of occurrences when a recipient had been in a coma whilst receiving distant healing. It was possible to elicit a meaningful response from that person that was to change the lives of their family and close friends.

It is also possible to transcend time, as well as space, using the distant healing method. Healing can therefore be sent backwards to a difficult period in your life or forward to an important time in the future. The results can be highly effective in bringing harmony to the present.

Absent healing can also be sent to situations as well as living beings and be transmitted to war zones or disaster areas throughout the world. There is a networking organisation called the Reiki Outreach International, founded by Mary McFadyen, an American Reiki Master, which co-ordinates the sending of energy to world situations, so that as much distance healing as possible reaches a particular area or situation. Further information can be found at www.annieo.com/reikioutreach

Distant healing can be used to treat plants and shrubs. Even gardens, parks or weakened groves of trees can be treated on a regular basis. Animals, small and large, can be treated using the distant healing method; it is especially useful in treating those animals that are not safe to approach physically.

Rooms can be cleansed energetically by using the symbols. Offices or kitchens can be treated to minimise the effects of emissions from electrical equipment. It is recommended that appliances connected to the electrical supply should be at least two metres (six feet) away from where you sleep. All electrical equipment should be switched off and unplugged when not in use as well. Food can be treated to enhance its nutritional content. Raw food contains live enzymes and a high degree of life force energy. Cooked and pre-packaged supermarket food carries far less energy and benefits considerably from being treated, though there is no substitute for fresh, home-made food. We recommend Leslie Kenton's books (see Further Reading, page 168) for a high-energy diet containing lots of fresh raw fruit and vegetables. The recipes look and taste marvellous and literally transform your energy levels and your waistline without depriving you of substantial meals.

Surprisingly, Reiki can even be sent to computers, cars and other machines, and it is fascinating to see how faulty equipment can sometimes respond. All manufactured materials were constructed from organic substances originally and can be treated with Reiki, although it would be unwise to depend on the results.

BEAMING REIKI ACROSS A ROOM

With Second Degree, you can beam Reiki across a room from your hands. This can be a useful technique, especially when it would not be appropriate to place hands on a person for any reason, for example if they are undergoing counselling. The distant healing method speeds up the counselling process and serves to help the person endure the emotional upheaval that may be surfacing.

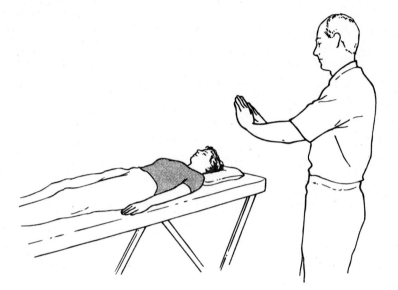

In conclusion, there are many ways in which distant healing can be used, some of which are mentioned above. Others are covered extensively in our Second Degree course. Two of these are described below.

THE REIKI BOX

An excellent way of sending absent healing to a number of people and situations at the same time is to use a Reiki box. This can be any kind of small box, ideally made of a natural material, such as wood. Place inside it either a photograph or simply the name of the persons or situations you would like to send Reiki to. You can even draw a simple picture or put a symbol in the box to represent who or what to send energy to. Draw the power symbols over each one as it is put into the box. (If you haven't taken Second Degree, simply place them in the box.) Holding the box, send absent healing to the contents. Do this on a regular basis, keeping the box solely for healing purposes, and the energy will accumulate, becoming more effective as it builds.

REIKI BANK

Another way of helping others is to open a Reiki 'bank account' for them. The idea of this is to send Reiki using the absent healing technique to their bank account so that they can draw on it whenever they need it. Simple and effective.

Second Degree and personal development

The Second Degree initiate can send Reiki to himself to heal old situations and pave the way energetically for those yet to come. It often happens that Second Degree initiates have overcome their initial fears and can move forward with a greater sense of wholeness and confidence than at First Degree level. There are also more energetic tools to work with at this level.

It becomes more important to decide what you would like to create in your life, how you wish to spend your time, who you wish to be with and which career would bring you the most fulfilment.

Thought is very powerful, and we are all constantly creating with the power of our thoughts. Whether it is planning the evening meal or deciding to enrol on a college course, it always begins with a thought. Negative thinking is draining and limiting. Positive thoughts are self-empowering and energising. Hence, worrying or holding a negative idea, such as illness, can eventually bring it about. Positive thinking is literally transformational. Choose to envisage yourself succeeding at whatever you set out to do and you will always be successful.

When making changes for ourselves, we create thoughts of new possibilities long before we take action. Energy is magnetic and tends to attract a similar vibration that is being radiated from elsewhere. This is why we often witness 'synchronicities' or 'coincidences'. An example of this is when the very person we have just been thinking about telephones us unexpectedly that same evening.

Discovering our dreams and making them happen isn't always easy and certainly requires some effort and dedication on our part. Once we ground our dreams and clarify our goals, we have the ability and the tools to manifest them. Our intentions are very powerful. Dr Deepak Chopra refers to our intent as 'the software of the mind'. All we need to do is to decide what we want, commit to it and then take action. If we simply think about something without setting our intent or committing to it, it becomes a whim. If we commit to it, we manifest it.

THE POWER OF FOCUS

It often happens in our everyday life that we have so many areas to give our attention to that we dissipate our energy and as a result lose the power of our focus. It is important to consolidate your focus and your attention. This is a major step in moving forwards and not becoming stuck from both an energetic and a practical point of view.

One person described suffering from constant exhaustion. She was surprised she didn't have any more energy, as her lifestyle was healthy and active. She went on to describe the many commodities and services she offered to others. The list was extensive. It included a dozen therapies, financial advice, picture framing, lecturing, printing, designing, writing, publishing and painting.

She was obviously a very capable, talented person. However, whilst talking about her life, she realised that if she decided to focus on fewer areas, she would conserve her energy and allow herself to progress at a steadier pace. Her energy would be focused in fewer directions, giving her more energy and vitality.

By concentrating on one or two major areas, it is possible to increase clarity and form a powerful personal vision that is easier for others to relate to. It's a question of choosing a path and then following it. You are always free to change and opt for a different path. It is difficult to follow all paths, especially at the same time.

Personal growth with Second Degree contains many possibilities and requires our focus, intent and commitment to bring about positive change. To be empowered, we need to have control over our lives and over our emotions, so that we can enjoy a greater sense of wholeness, harmony and balance.

In conclusion, the minimum requirements for the Usui System of Reiki at Second Degree are:

Nine hours' tuition
One initiation or attunement
Three symbols
Three mantras
Using the symbols
Distance healing
Mental and emotional healing

CHAPTER SEVEN

Master Practitioner

THIS COURSE WAS DEVELOPED in order to distinguish between vocational teachers of Reiki and those wishing to attain the highest level of practitioner skills. This distinction clarifies whether or not a person has been trained as a teaching Master. The word 'master' is used in the Eastern sense, referring to someone who teaches but who focuses more on mastering self than being a master of others. Traditionally, it has often been used as a term of deference in areas such as martial arts training, yoga and Zen Buddhism. The term 'Master Practitioner' in relation to Reiki denotes a person whose focus is on reaching high levels mentally and spiritually in order to use energy healing in a way that most benefits others.

Training at this level involves finding out who you really are. We are often keen to help others without really dealing with our own issues. It is about being able to completely accept yourself, without being limited by the ego's illusory messages.

We always advise students considering training at this level to leave a gap of at least six months between Reiki Second Degree and Master Practitioner. This is so that they can assimilate and practise the material learned earlier. Many prefer to wait longer, until they are sure they are ready to take the next step.

Not every Master offers this course. We feel it is an important step for those who are considering the possibility of training as a teaching Master, as well as for those who wish to practise at the highest level.

Following this training, many find it becomes easier to move beyond limiting thought patterns. Once you are able to do this, it is easier to help others to do so. You may also find that the knowledge and energetic boost at Master Practitioner level allows you to take a more active role in creating your own experience.

Whilst the course focuses largely on self-mastery, students also learn some powerful techniques for healing and transformation. These vary. The following techniques are taught by some Reiki Masters (although not necessarily by ourselves) and are examples of the sort of exercises often taught on courses at this level.

CANDLE·FLAME TECHNIQUE

This is an interesting absent healing technique. It involves using the flame of a candle or an oil lamp to represent the people or situations that will receive the energy. Write out a list of everyone and everything you wish to send energy to. Then place the list underneath a candle or oil lamp. Light it and set the intent that the flame represents the list, and that as long as the flame burns, the list and everyone and everything on it will receive an individual, complete and continuous Reiki treatment. Then, using the absent healing technique learned at Reiki Second Degree, use the symbols to set up an energetic pathway and start the healing process.

CONTINUOUSLY RESONATING FIELD OF REIKI ENERGY

- Choose four similarly sized crystals. Cleanse all the crystals in sea salt and distilled or purified water for a period of twenty-four hours or more.
- Pick up each crystal and draw the three Second Degree symbols on each. Empower each one with the following intentions: (a) That they are to be used for healing purposes for an infinite number of Reiki treatments; (b) That they are activated whenever the molecules in the crystals move or vibrate. Place an unlimited supply of power symbols within each one.

- Place the four crystals either in the corners of a room, on the outside corners of a house or building or on the boundaries of a garden.
- Visualise the energy fields connecting all four crystals, creating an energy field that continues upward above the ground, as well as downward beneath the ground.
- Draw or visualise the symbols in the direction of the resonating field of energy, and empower the enclosed space with unlimited power symbols.
- Repeat the intent that the resonating field of Reiki energy continues its action with each molecular vibration.
- Everything within the space of the crystals will continue to receive an on-going treatment of Reiki. You might even do this around your own bed. It should help you to sleep and remain more relaxed and healthy.

MANIFESTING GOALS WITH REIKI

Sit and relax, breathing gently and deeply. Either in your mind or aloud, say your goal. Phrase it simply and clearly. Connect to the Reiki energy using the method learned at Second Degree. Visualise this goal being attained. Draw the Reiki symbols on the picture you have envisaged, starting and ending with the power symbol. Repeat this procedure for each goal you wish to accomplish. Finish by drawing all the Reiki symbols again on the visualisation and sealing it with a power symbol. Believe totally that this process is complete and this goal has already been manifested.

Master Practitioner is an advanced training and doesn't necessarily follow a fixed format. Whilst students usually receive a Master level symbol and attunement, the remaining material will usually be tailored to meet the needs of the particular group. It often opens the door to a new higher path, and when taught well, it accelerates a person's self-development and lays a solid foundation for spiritual growth towards self-mastery.

CHAPTER EIGHT

Reiki Master Teacher

MASTER TEACHER IS FOR those wishing to help others become channels for Reiki energy. We recommend that anyone wishing to undertake this training allows a gap of around twelve months from taking Second Degree training. This is to integrate the energies and gain adequate experience of using the material, to be able to competently assist others to benefit from its practice.

Traditionally this path is seen as a calling, and at the time of Dr Usui, a person who wished to become a Reiki Master would serve as an apprentice until Dr Usui felt that they were ready to be initiated as a Master in their own right.

Today there are a variety of Masters' trainings available in the West. Some offer brief courses with little or no teacher training. Others are lengthier, with opportunities to take part in future seminars and even co-teach until a person feels confident enough to hold their own classes. There is also a longer, apprenticeship-style training, such as Dr Usui offered. All have advantages and disadvantages.

At the very minimum, courses include an initiation, a symbol, some healing techniques and a course manual. Many taking this type of training do not intend to teach Reiki anyway and the content is probably sufficient for their personal use. Those who do intend to teach would be wise to seek out a teacher who can provide more.

The Reiki Alliance, an organisation formed following the death of Mrs Takata, honours the traditional training by insisting that all its members train future Masters using the apprenticeship approach.

This route is quite expensive, as Mrs Takata equated the cost of training to the level of the trainee's personal commitment. In its favour, it must be said that the cost of spiritual and personal growth is difficult to quantify in our consumer-oriented society. It must also be taken into account that this type of training is personalised, being tailored to the individual needs of the student. Trainees certainly receive sufficient grounding and plenty of practice. There is also enough time for the student to gain a good understanding of the material and to benefit from personalised coaching.

This kind of training is extremely helpful to someone intending to teach. What you are really paying for is someone to train you to understand your own processes so clearly that you can shine a torch for others to pave the way for their journeys. If your own understanding and experience is superficial, limited or misguided, it does not bode well for future students. It may be possible to deceive your training Master over a short period of time, but you wouldn't delude future students for long. If only a few months are invested in your own personal development, there is no guarantee that you will have evolved sufficiently to master your own inner processes, let alone be in a position to guide others. There is no substitute for experience gained over a longer period with a skilled Reiki Master. Find someone who can train you well, plus guide and support you later when you begin to teach.

To conclude, there are many different courses available. It is possible to buy the title of Master via the briefest of courses, but for those who truly wish to be a Master, a high degree of personal responsibility is needed, as well as a correspondingly high level of commitment. In our opinion, there needs to be a lengthier training than just two days, if you are intending to teach. Experience is required before we gain enough understanding to assist others. A wise sage cannot compile all his knowledge and understanding into a manual and ask someone else to take his place, because they simply won't be able to.

There are many shorter courses to choose from today; however, there are fewer Masters offering an apprenticeship-style route. For those considering this training, it is important to find a teacher that you resonate with, as you will be spending time with this person and need to establish a good rapport at the outset.

Whatever training is taken, the student should have progressed sufficiently to be thirsting for more knowledge by the end of the course. The trainee should be willing, flexible and disciplined enough to progress down a path of continuous self-development with a clearer personal vision of his or her future and the ability to be able to create it.

As the length of each course differs, so do the contents. As a rule, students are initiated and learn how to attune others. They receive the Master symbol. We know Dr Usui greatly valued this symbol and felt it to be sacred and powerful. Some Reiki Masters suggest that students use it only occasionally, when something special is called for, or when they intuitively feel it is needed. Today, many teachers take a more liberal view of its use and use attunements as a 'booster' or energetic 'tune-up'. This is entirely up to the individual. Many use their intuition to know what feels right for them.

PERSONAL COACHING

Some Master Teaching training, especially the apprenticeship type, offers personal coaching as well. This usually focuses on issues appropriate to the student in order to further their self-development and provide opportunity for spiritual growth.

The need for clarity and understanding of the spiritual and mystical nature of the initiations and the profound changes that can occur is an important aspect of this work. It is also important for the student to understand the limitations of the energy and hold a realistic understanding of what it can and cannot do.

Some Masters give practical assistance and advice, such as in the setting up and running of a successful healing centre. Ideally, this should include financial and marketing guidelines as well as practice management.

Overall, it is important for the student to have a full understanding of the Reiki healing system, as well as a grounding in psychotherapy and esoteric knowledge. To continue the tradition as a Master and impart it to others requires a number of abilities. One would need to have the stability to hold a high level of energy consistently and observe the whole experience with a measure of humility, reverence and humour. Humour is an essential part of the process, to prevent a person from becoming self-centred or taking themselves too seriously.

Many Masters offer well-rounded training and support afterwards (further information in Chapter Nine). Recommendation and the Internet are good places to start looking.

How to Find a Reiki Master

REIKI IS EASY TO LEARN, and there are now Reiki Masters teaching in or near major cities in many parts of the world. The demand for Reiki training has risen substantially over the past ten years, and whilst there is some excellent tuition available, it has to be said that training as a whole is variable. However, it is not quite such a minefield if you are willing to invest a small amount of time and effort to assess whether the tuition offered is of a high standard.

Reiki is an oral tradition and initiations or attunements should be carried out face-to-face with a Reiki Master, usually in a group setting. Anyone offering attunements by mail, telephone, the Internet, a book, or even from a different room is not providing adequate Reiki training and should not even be considered. This is different from sending or receiving absent healing, which, of course, can be done from across the world.

The size of the group is important, as each participant should receive personal attention and support. In very large groups, unless there are a number of Reiki Masters or teaching assistants present, the needs of the individual may be overlooked.

We are all individual and there are bound to be considerable variations in the way each teacher imparts the same knowledge to students. Mrs Takata taught Reiki as an intuitive healing art and not a rigid system as such. However, a good teacher should be able to demonstrate that they offer a high standard of training. This should include individual attention during courses and support afterwards.

The Usui System of Reiki is complete and does not require extra initiations or levels to improve or enhance it in any way. It is a system that imparts sacred knowledge and energetic attunement to allow healing ability to be initiated and personal growth to be accelerated, both at the time and over a period of many years to come.

Even though it appears to be a simple form of hands-on healing, Reiki is still a path of initiation and consequently a mystic tradition. It is important to find a person you trust and who has the experience to provide guidance and empathy to allow you to understand and appreciate the vastness of Reiki.

Whilst finding the right Reiki Master can sometimes appear a daunting task, it is helpful to remember that the best way to find a teacher is often through the personal endorsement of others. Many advertisements only contain a name and the date of classes and it is not possible to find out what sort of tuition is being offered. Also, the best teachers sometimes never advertise at all. Where possible, make personal contact with the person, assess what kind of classes are being offered and then go with your inner feelings, trusting that you are making the right decision. It is far better to wait a little longer for the right teacher than to take the first opportunity offered, which might feel wrong at the outset.

It helps greatly if you feel you have rapport with the teacher. Ask yourself whether you think this Master could impart information to you in a meaningful way. Courses are experiential rather than theoretical. It is important to find someone whom you feel you could trust to provide the right environment for you to grow and develop. As a culture, we have a tendency to complicate things. A good teacher will help you to strip away the layers of anger, pain, etc., and connect with the simplicity of Reiki.

Avoid anyone who pressures you to make a decision about taking a place on a course. Ask yourself if you feel the Master is a well-balanced person who is comfortable to be with. Should a teacher show you disrespect in any way, look elsewhere. Beware of Masters who have only taken the briefest of training with little experience themselves. Everyone has to start somewhere, but a Master who has real commitment to Reiki will have practised for a number of years before taking Master Teacher training, and will have a track record going back further than just last week.

People vary, but generally speaking a good teacher should have a pleasant, joyful disposition with good humour. You should feel comfortable and at peace in their presence. Notice if they are sincere or somewhat overly impressed by all the people they have healed. A genuine Reiki Master will never proselytise or make claims which sound too good to be true.

Impressive degrees, titles or certificates on the wall do not necessarily signify a well-balanced person. Common sense and depth of experience is more important. Ask yourself how that person makes you feel about yourself. Do you feel good about yourself in their presence?

Recommendation and direct contact is one of the best ways of finding a Reiki Master. If you do not know anyone who has taken Reiki training, start by contacting national or international complementary therapy organisations. There are also Reiki Master associations in most countries, which list their members. A list and details of websites can be found at the back of the book.

Avoid making decisions based on convenience. There may be excellent Reiki Masters in your locality, but it may be better to travel a little further for the right teacher than to make a mistake closer to home.

part three

HEALING
WITH
REIKI

CHAPTER TEN

Reiki Treatments

Experiencing a Reiki treatment

REIKI HAS GROWN TREMENDOUSLY in popularity and treatments are now widely available at nearly every holistic clinic, spa or complementary medicine centre in Britain, Europe, the USA, Australia and many other countries worldwide. Many practitioners work from home or offer treatments at locations to suit the client.

Reactions to treatment vary considerably from person to person. The most common element experienced is one of deep relaxation and a feeling of warmth in particular areas of the body. Some people experience tingling, vibration, warmth, cool areas, twitches, crying, laughter and stomach rumblings. Sometimes it is possible to become aware of an old wound as the scar tissue receives healing. Occasionally a brief discomfort is felt for a short while. This is unusual. It is more typical to experience a blissful, euphoric feeling that enables you to sink into a deep state of relaxation.

It is usual to lie down for a full treatment, as the individual will often drift off or fall into a 'Reiki slumber', as we have come to name it. Treatment is no less effective when the recipient has slept through it entirely. It may be just what is required.

Following treatment, many people feel rather dreamy and relaxed and may need to sit down for a while to become grounded again before leaving.

It is recommended that at least one glass of water is drunk

following treatment, as toxins are loosened that need flushing through the system. Ideally, liquid intake, preferably water, should be increased considerably over the 24–48-hour period following treatment. This is for two reasons. First, it prevents headaches caused by the presence of any toxins remaining in the system. Second, the energy can make you very thirsty and it would not be helpful to become dehydrated.

It is inadvisable to drink alcohol for at least twenty-four hours after receiving Reiki, as it could have an undesirable effect on a delicate system undergoing detoxification. Depending on a person's well-being at the time, it is recommended that an initial course of three to four treatments is booked, rather than just one. The effects are cumulative and it is highly likely that several treatments will be needed to complete the healing process. For pain relief, for example, one session will probably relieve the discomfort, but several will enable the energy to reach the causal level of the problem and prevent further occurrences. Discomfort may be caused by tension held in a particular area where the individual has internalised something going on in their life. Someone declaring they 'can't stomach a situation' may find they suffer a stomach disorder as a result of internalising the problem. Reiki may provide insight as to the cause of such a complaint. Such insight can cause the symptom to be quickly relieved.

The energy always goes to the causal level, not necessarily to the symptom. Whilst it is highly likely that the symptom will be relieved by the treatment, healing at a causal level will have undoubtedly taken place. If, for example, a person is extremely tense, it is possible that the tension has been internalised, and has subsequently manifested itself as a physical problem somewhere in the body. If the treatment releases the tension and even gives insight as to where the problem originated, it can highlight areas where the person needs to make lifestyle changes.

Insights as to the causes of symptoms are not uncommon during a Reiki session. One of our clients had suffered from constipation for most of her life. Over the years, she had tried many orthodox medicines, herbal remedies and a number of complementary therapies without success. Before the treatment started, we suggested that she allow herself to understand why she had this disorder. As soon as this session finished, she became anxious to share her experience. She described a scene that had unfolded in her mind during the treatment, which clarified why she had suffered so long.

As a child during the Second World War, she had been sent to stay with an aunt in the country. Although it happened a long time ago, she was able to recall the surroundings clearly, even remembering the dress her aunt was wearing. She was also able to clearly remember that the toilet was situated across a yard in the back garden. It turned out that she had been severely punished on more than one occasion for using far too much toilet paper at a time when such commodities were very scarce. As soon as she realised that it was the fear of punishment so long ago that had caused her to become constipated, she was very pleased to have reached the root of the problem. She knew that this would never bother her again and disposed of her medicines on the way out.

For further information about the metaphysical causes of specific individual symptoms, read Louise Hay's book *Heal Your Body*.

Not all insights highlight the cause of a symptom. Some reveal the solution. One person who came for a treatment had an insight that was to change his life. He was a family man who had been extremely wealthy. Due to some poor business decisions, a crooked business partner and the effects of the recession, he had lost everything, including his home. He was not usually interested in complementary therapies of any sort, but as he had lapsed into a deep depression and was almost suicidal, we offered him a treatment to see if it would help at all.

Uncharacteristically, he accepted and duly arrived for his first session. His self-esteem was very low and he hardly spoke before the session. He slept deeply throughout his first treatment and told us afterwards that it was the first time he had relaxed for many months. He came back for several more sessions.

During what was to be the final session, he described receiving inspiration that was to bring considerable positive change. Despite having no money, no home and no hope of receiving financial backing of any kind, he knew he must return to the industry where he had started as a young man. He had received an idea during his Reiki treatment that would enable him to supply a product to a unique outlet. He decided that he would immediately start another business. He knew it would not be easy, having learned many lessons from his previous enterprise. It was difficult for him to re-establish himself and he overcame many obstacles that would have deterred others. Happily, his determination has resulted in him being able to earn a living once more and successfully provide for his family.

The healing process

Sometimes, during treatment, just as progress has been made, it is possible for a healing crisis to occur, which can bring about the return of all the original symptoms. This is a natural part of the healing process for some people. It can, though, be an unexpectedly traumatic experience for the person being treated and usually indicates that deeply repressed emotions have surfaced. However, it is comforting to know that the symptoms are not back to stay.

Such a crisis can occur because of the acceleration in the course of the illness. Other healing crises may feature uncontrollable crying or even an unexpected skin rash emerging. These usually pass quickly and are no cause for concern. Of course, it is necessary to have healing and support during this until the symptoms diminish.

Reactions to treatment vary enormously and results are unpredictable. The gentle healing energy is always drawn by the person receiving the treatment and usually at the pace that suits their system. In a sense all healing is self-healing; the healer is simply providing the right conditions for healing to occur. It is then up to the recipient. After several Reiki sessions, it is usual to feel energised, positive and pain free, with plenty of confidence and enthusiasm.

We are often asked the cost of a Reiki treatment. This varies enormously. As a rule, it is usually equivalent to the cost of a body massage in your area. Practitioners can usually be found at complementary medicine centres, health spas or holistic beauty salons. Otherwise, the Internet can be a useful resource, or see the Useful Websites section at the back of the book.

Self-healing

Most participants on our training courses tell us that they enrolled principally because they wish to use Reiki to treat themselves. Self-treatment is very simple and effective as a means of relaxation and stress relief. Sufferers from fatigue syndromes often find they have raised energy levels after experiencing Reiki. Hyperactivity is usually tempered by deep relaxation after taking Reiki and emotional balance is restored. Reiki often relieves pain from acute conditions, though chronic conditions can take longer and may spark a healing crisis before symptoms diminish fully.

Twenty-one-day energy integration

During Reiki training, it is suggested that a full self-treatment is given for at least twenty-one days. There are four main reasons for this:

- Daily self-treatment is the fastest way to integrate the increased energy into an individual's system. Daily treatment allows the energy to move strongly into the physical body to bring about physiological changes. It allows the balancing and integrating of emotional, mental and spiritual bodies.
- A self-cleanse mechanism is triggered by the attunements and the system starts to detoxify. Self-treatment assists this process.
- Before giving Reiki to others, it is necessary to heal ourselves. Receiving the energy on a daily basis in this way facilitates the start of our own healing.
- You are likely to become far more aware of the energy flow during a concentrated period of self-treatment. Additionally, it will be easier to notice the effect on others.

Most people find they thoroughly enjoy making time for these nurturing sessions and continue them long after the recommended period has elapsed, making them part of their daily routine. Others find they initially encounter some less pleasant reactions. It is not unheard of to experience mild diarrhoea or sickness following training. This is usually because of detoxification. Very occasionally, a rash could appear on the skin. Healing always begins within and moves outwards to the surface of the body. Such a rash would not be a cause for concern and would usually indicate that healing and cleansing are occurring.

Sometimes it happens that strong emotions begin to surface during the twenty-one-day cleansing period. This can happen at any time thereafter. The energy provides strength to deal with any fear or other emotions that appear, and we always suggest persevering with self-treatment as they rapidly diminish. Should there be issues surfacing that are difficult to deal with on one's own, it may be helpful to arrange to see a suitable therapist who can provide the necessary support and assistance on a one-to-one basis.

Treating yourself: the twelve basic positions

Below is a guide to self-treatment, which is ideal for those who have taken Reiki First Degree training. A self-treatment CD is available from The Reiki School to accompany self-treatments; details can be found on page 164. People who haven't taken Reiki training can follow and benefit from the positions shown as well; however, the attunements received during training will substantially increase the energy flow and make quite a difference to the session.

Lie down and allow yourself to become relaxed and comfortable. It is suggested when giving yourself a Reiki treatment that you stay in each position for five minutes, which means that you will spend about an hour on a full treatment using all twelve positions.

FIRST POSITION

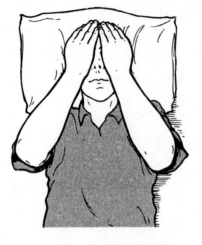

With your fingers closed and the hands slightly cupped, move to the first position over the eyes. Allow the hands to remain still with a light touch whilst they are placed in the various holds. Practice will determine a touch that is not too light, nor too heavy. At a physical level the energy transmission in this position affects the pituitary and pineal glands, as well as the eyes, sinuses, nose, teeth and jaws. At an emotional level, it helps to reduce stress. At a mental level, this position helps the process of thought and concentration, increases clarity and improves decision-making. It is also the natural position used to treat a headache. In the Bates method of natural healing, it is suggested that this position is maintained for up to an hour a day to improve vision.

This position also assists in awakening the third eye, a term which many forms of Eastern medicine use to refer to the part of us where mental pictures are formed and where our intuition or inspiration is drawn from. There are forms of healing that work solely towards awakening the third eye, as they feel that when it is activated and awakened, it enables the person to see the God or Divine within everyone and everything, allowing a state of harmony at all levels to be experienced. The third eye is said to give inner sight where it is possible to see auras and energy.

You may feel heat in your hands which may seem to turn on and then, when you have been in this position for a while, diminish and appear to switch off. This is a natural regulating process and happens when the body no longer needs the energy in a particular position and either reduces or simply stops it altogether.

SECOND POSITION

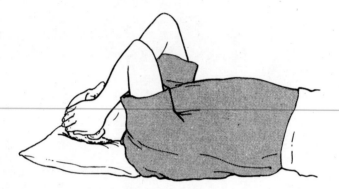

Without lifting them off the body, move the hands to second position over the temples. At a physical level, this position affects the brain. As the Reiki energy begins to flow into the temple areas of the head, it promotes the release of any mental tension and gradually calms the mind whilst slowing the brain's activity. It is good for headaches and seizures, as well as the pituitary and pineal glands. It assists with shock and motion sickness.

At an emotional level, it works to help relieve worry, hysteria, stress and depression. This position helps to enhance dream recall. At a mental level, it assists in creating calmness, and helps to improve memory retention, productivity and creativity.

Whilst in this position, the energy helps to awaken and activate the crown chakra. Chakras are an Eastern concept and refer to the various points over certain parts of the body through which energy passes. Chakras are seen as rotating wheels or spinning cones of light within the energy field or aura surrounding the body. Energy is able to pass through the chakras and enter the body. For detailed information about the function of chakras, see Chapter Eleven. The crown chakra is said to be the connection to cosmic information. It is the link to one's higher self.

As the Reiki energy flows through a person in the first and second positions, it helps to integrate the right and left hemispheres of the brain. The left brain is the logical, analytical part that works with mathematics, for example. The right brain is the intuitive, receptive, imaginative part. The language of the right brain is symbols. The right and left brain also contain the feminine and masculine aspects of the body, known as yin and yang. When the energies between the two sides of the brain are balanced, it is possible for a person to be more flexible and to use whatever mode is appropriate for a situation. It is easier to effectively create the situations that are desired in one's life.

THIRD POSITION

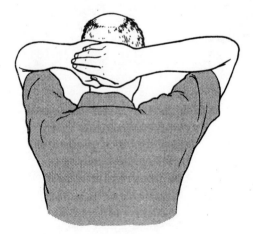

The third position, with your hands at the back of your head, at the base of your skull and over the occipital lobe, affects weight and vision. It assists with speech and controls the nervous system for the entire body. At an emotional level, it releases stress and promotes relaxation. It relieves pain and enhances dream and past life recall. At a mental level, it calms thoughts and helps relieve depression. This position is one where a mother holds a new baby before it is strong enough to hold its own head up. This is a very nurturing and supportive position for yourself (and for others).

This area affects the will-centre, and when this centre is constricted you are likely to give your power away to others and not see your own value and worthiness. It is one of the places that tend to absorb a great deal of energy. There is a need to stay balanced in this area, so that maximum performance may occur.

FOURTH POSITION

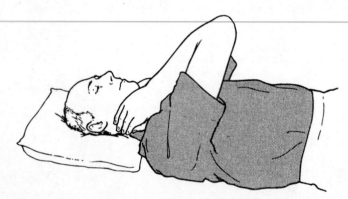

The fourth position is over the throat and jawline. At a physical level the energy assists with strokes, tonsils, throat, larynx, thyroid and parathyroid and helps in balancing blood pressure both high and low. This position improves lymphatic drainage.

At a mental level, this position brings calmness and clarity of thought. At an emotional level, it helps to bring confidence and joy, as well as to relieve anger, hostility and resentment. The jaw is one of the places where we store a tremendous amount of emotion. In this area we often hold on to feelings of old rage, helplessness and anger. As a culture we have a great fear of speaking our truth. We tend to swallow our words rather than speak them in anger or share them. As the energy moves into this part of the body, it begins to activate the throat. It may be felt as a 'pins and needles' sensation, or you may feel you want to clear your throat or cough. That's usually a good indication that there has been some holding back, that words have not been spoken.

As the energy balances this part of the body, it becomes much easier for a person to speak freely. Every word is an expression of who that person is, and every time an individual does not speak their truth, it has an effect upon their physiological system and upon that person's life.

FIFTH POSITION

The fifth position is over the heart. At a physical level, this treats the heart, lungs and thymus and affects the immune system and circulation. At an emotional level it facilitates the release of stress and assists in enhancing the capacity to love and be loved. At a mental level it helps to restore balance and harmony.

As you work with yourself and others, you begin to discover that everyone has heart issues. As a culture we have learned to protect our hearts, to not allow love in or out. We have figuratively built walls of protection around the heart. As the Reiki energy moves into this area, it begins to take those walls down, block by block. There are times when it is possible to feel physical movement in this part of the body.

Whilst in this position, and as the blocks are being removed, it is possible to find the circulation of blood is affected, allowing a greater flow throughout the body. As the energy moves into and through this area, there may be vibrations, tremors or spasms. Again, this is releasing the blocks of those walls and allowing one's heart to function in a natural state of harmony. Bringing energy into this part of the body allows you to truly experience the emotional self.

SIXTH POSITION

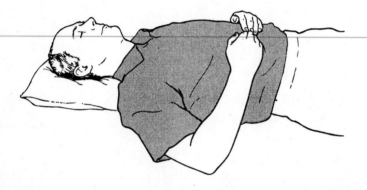

The sixth position, just below the chest but still on the rib cage, is over the solar plexus area. At a physical level, this affects the liver, stomach, spleen, gall bladder and digestion. At an emotional level it brings relaxation and helps to release fears and stress. At a mental level it helps to centre oneself.

The solar plexus is our point of power in the body. It is that part that martial arts instructors teach you to draw from and to protect. When somebody hurts you, it can feel as if they have punched you in the stomach. You may feel helpless, unprotected, as if you have no power. Your confidence can be shattered, you may doubt yourself and feel hesitant to act. When this area is in balance, you feel confident, secure and strong, able to move forward with ease. There is a stream of energy that comes up from your base chakra, at your tailbone, moving up through your solar plexus. When this energy flows freely, it helps to develop greater self-confidence. The energy stream continues up through the heart, bringing love and compassion. Simultaneously there is a stream of energy that comes down through the top of your head, through the crown chakra, bringing in wisdom. It allows you to be all that you can be, in balance and in love. As the energy moves through the entire body, it brings unity within.

SEVENTH POSITION

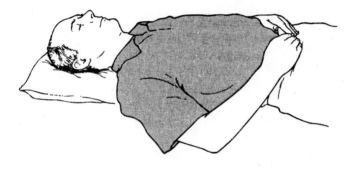

The seventh position is over the abdomen. At a physical level it affects the liver, pancreas, gall bladder and transverse colon. At an emotional level it affects issues of bitterness, fault-finding, negative feelings and frustration. This centre processes the sweets of life. Diabetes is a disease that does not allow one to properly digest sweets. The gall bladder relates to bitterness, as obliquely referred to in the expression 'of all the gall'. This is the centre wherein angry thoughts and words are held, creating feelings of bitterness, blame and frustration.

Bringing energy to this area assists in releasing negative thoughts and gives us an opportunity to realise that we create our own lives. We use experiences simply to learn, and clearing this area provides us with the gift of learning and growing from situations around us. It also facilitates our digestion of the sweeter emotions, such as harmony and joy. Treatment in this position is very calming. Using the energy, it brings balance and alignment of the physical, emotional and mental bodies, simultaneously bringing harmony at all levels.

EIGHTH POSITION

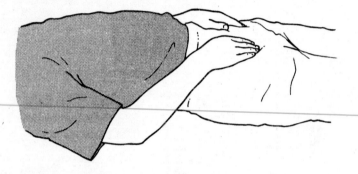

The eighth position is over the pelvic area. At a physical level, this affects lymphatic drainage and the release of toxins. It affects the large and small intestines, the bladder, issues of constipation and diarrhoea, and the ovaries, uterus and prostate. At an emotional level, this centre relates to feelings of security and pleasure. At a mental level it is the area of creativity and elimination, of pleasure and creativity and letting go of unneeded, outdated ideas and substances.

This is the place from which we express our sexual ecstasy and pleasure, sexual frustration and guilt, and resentment of our partner or our parent of the opposite sex. As physical, mental and emotional issues come into our awareness, it is important to remember that this is also the centre where we release ideas and thoughts that no longer serve our highest good. We are able to replace them with feelings and thoughts that can assist us to fully and joyfully express all aspects of ourselves.

NINTH POSITION

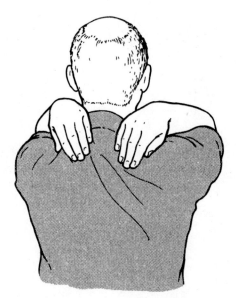

This position is at the top of the shoulders. The four back positions have a similar purpose to the four front positions. At a physical level, this position affects the heart as well as the shoulders and the neck. At an emotional level it facilitates the release of stress and burdens. At a mental level it brings peace and harmony. This is the area where most of us experience tension, giving rise to the feelings that we're carrying the weight of the world on our shoulders.

It is possible in stressful situations to briefly place your hands on your shoulders and take a few long, slow, deep breaths. At the same time it is helpful to remind yourself to relax, whilst becoming aware of the energy as it moves in, feeling all the positive aspects of the experience as you release any tension.

TENTH POSITION

The tenth position is over the shoulder blades. This position affects the heart and the lungs at a physical level. At an emotional

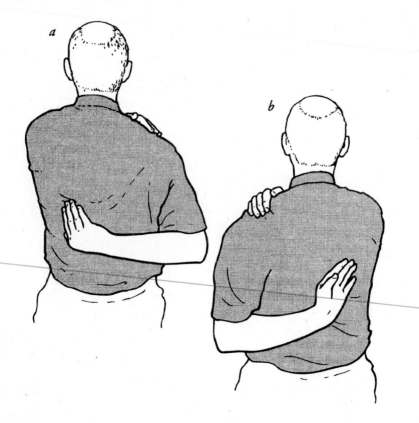

level it enhances the ability to love and be loved, as well as facilitating the release of stress. At a mental level, this position brings peace and harmony. Positions (a) and (b) show handholds to treat both sides of the shoulder blades. When spending five minutes in the other positions, allow two and a half minutes each in 10a and 10b.

ELEVENTH POSITION

The eleventh position is over the lower back. At a physical level, this affects the gall bladder, pancreas and transverse colon, as well as the adrenal glands, the kidneys and the lower back. At an emotional

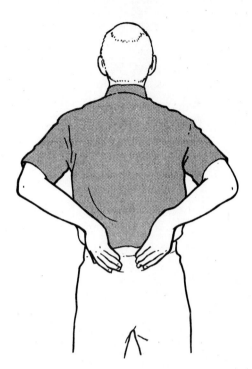

level it assists in releasing self-criticism, anxiety and negativity. This, again, is the area in which we hold feelings such as negativity, blaming and fault-finding. When we choose to release old feelings and thoughts, we create space for more positive emotions, such as harmony and joy. Life becomes much lighter and clearer and we experience situations in a more positive way.

When there is a pain in the physical body, it can sometimes be recognised as a bell ringing. It may help to ask what is going on in this area. Pain may suggest there is resistance in the body; perhaps some emotion or feeling has been suppressed. When there is pain, simply begin by focusing your attention on it and asking 'What is my body saying to me?' or 'What is it I need to be aware of?'

The body can be likened to a projection screen on to which our emotions and thoughts are projected. At a physical level, we tend to pay attention, whereas we dismiss our thoughts and emotions all too easily. So, when we have a pain in the body and we recognise that there is something out of order, it can assist us to become aware of what the cause is. Our bodies are wonderful instruments that notify us and allow us to bring disharmony into conscious awareness, so that we can begin to acknowledge and deal with the real issues and causes behind the discomfort or pain.

TWELFTH POSITION

This is over the tailbone. Physically this affects the large and small intestines, bladder, uterus, ovaries, prostate and coccyx. At an emotional and mental level it is the centre of creativity and releasing. This is the seat of our power from where we create and release our desires and responses. When we hold on to old feelings

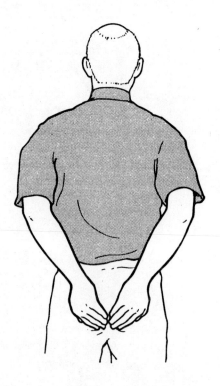

or responses, we tend to concentrate on them and not make room for new ideas. Releasing old thoughts and feelings makes room for new innovative and creative expressions. When this happens we are reaching true expressions of our potential, to become all that we can be.

Energy goes to where it is needed. Once connected to the energy, each person's evolutionary progression is encouraged. Focus is drawn to the expression of loving, positive emotions such as caring, nurturing, compassion, trusting and self-acceptance.

Healing others

(For details of hand positions, see Chapter Five)

A typical treatment will last for about an hour. In the case of children or someone physically frail, a twenty-minute treatment is often sufficient. It is usual to give a Reiki treatment whilst the client is lying down in a comfortable position, although if this is not possible for any reason, it can be given sitting up in a chair or in whichever position the client is comfortable.

Giving five minutes in each position is a good guide. If the person you are working with has a number of severe symptoms, you will want to treat them as much as five times in the first week, four times in the next, three the next, two the next, and then once a week for several weeks thereafter to give them optimum availability of the energy. If you are not able to do this, then perhaps you can give them three Reiki treatments the first week, two the next and once a week for several weeks thereafter. It is beneficial to allow a person to receive maximum exposure to the energy, because the cumulative effect helps to bring results that are more positive.

If their symptoms are more than minor, it is of course essential for them to be referred to their own medical practitioner for treatment besides receiving Reiki.

When time is limited

Short treatments are sometimes appropriate depending on the situation. Someone suffering from a headache can find that relief is obtained by receiving Reiki in just two or three head positions, whilst sitting upright in a chair. In an emergency, a short Reiki treatment is ideal whilst waiting for help to arrive. If a person tends to have particularly strong reactions or has powerful build-ups of energy, then again, short treatments would be preferable initially.

Short treatments may also be appropriate if someone is in considerable pain or discomfort and cannot remain still for any length of time. In the case of someone suffering from a particularly severe complaint, it might be wiser to initially avoid the problem area, allowing the energy to flow through other areas to rebalance and strengthen the system. Small children neither need nor appreciate lengthy treatments. Animals tend to let us know when they have had enough.

Usui Reiki teaches twelve basic hand positions that cover the major parts of the body; however, there are infinitely more positions that can be used depending on the situation.

PREPARATION

The room in which a treatment is to be given needs to be warm as well as in a quiet location. The person receiving the treatment will usually be lying down, ideally on a treatment couch, although any sufficiently long oblong table (such as a dining table) will suffice.

It may be helpful to cover the person with a light blanket to ensure they do not become too cool during the treatment. If the sunlight is strong, it may be preferable to draw the blinds or curtains, although this is not essential. Some practitioners choose to play background music, usually with tranquil, non-intrusive sounds, such as music reflecting a natural forest or the sound of water flowing. If you choose to have background music playing, select the repeat function, so that it does not end suddenly during treatment. Switch on the answering machine and disconnect the telephone, or at least reduce its volume to prevent the person and yourself being startled during a treatment. The practitioner needs to be as comfortable as possible, and may choose to be seated for as many of the positions as possible. A chair on wheels for the practitioner will allow easy movement from one position to another.

An illuminated clock is invaluable to watch the time spent in each position, although it is now possible to buy various music albums especially composed for Reiki treatments, with background bells indicating when to move on to the next position (see page 164). Scented oil burners with essential oils, such as lavender diluted in water, will help to create a pleasant, soothing atmosphere, although care should be taken when placing these in the room to ensure they are safely positioned.

Before beginning a treatment, spend a few moments with the client to welcome them and to ascertain why they have come for a Reiki treatment. Explain what Reiki is, what will happen over the next hour or so, to put them at ease and give them an idea of what they may expect. Ideally, the practitioner's hands should be washed before and again after the treatment. When the treatment has concluded, both the healer and the person receiving the treatment should drink a full glass of water. This assists the treatment by facilitating the toxic clearout.

SETTING THE INTENT

Just before the treatment begins, it is a good idea to suggest that the person decides where they would like the energy to go in their lives. This only takes a moment and need not be spoken aloud. The energy may be directed to a physical pain, to enhance emotional well-being or perhaps to a particular relationship or career path. All that is necessary is to close the eyes and quietly say, 'I would like the energy to go to . . .' and then list as many areas and situations as desired. Once the intent has been set, the person should be guided to relax and enjoy the treatment. It isn't necessary to concentrate on the choice after setting the intent. Wherever it is directed, the energy will then flow.

Before placing the hands in the first position, the practitioner briefly scans the body with their hands a few centimetres above the client. This is to ascertain which areas particularly need the energy. By using the hands to sense where the energy is required, the practitioner has a guide and can focus on particular areas accordingly. It may be necessary to spend more time in one area, especially if it is a specified requirement of the person being treated.

RECOMMENDATIONS FOR TREATMENT

During treatment, comfort and relaxation are paramount. It is also important to follow carefully the guidelines given in the Reiki training class. Make sure you tilt your head to one side whilst treating the head positions, so that you are not breathing over the person lying on the couch. Ensure you have not eaten excessively strong-smelling or spicy foods before giving a treatment. It is also vital to position your hands carefully so that they do not come into contact with the client's nose, mouth or throat at any time. The person being treated will then be able to relax completely, without feeling their breathing is being restricted in any way.

Your hands should be relaxed and slightly arched; your fingers should be kept together and applied without pressure to the body. The treatment can be given without physical contact, a few centimetres off the body, if either the practitioner or the person receiving the treatment prefers that. It is important to avoid hovering so lightly that it is barely felt on the body, as this can be a little disconcerting and rather off-putting for the client. We prefer to work on the body, as we feel that our society has little enough physical contact. A Reiki treatment should provide a secure, non-threatening and nurturing experience.

It will be natural to give Reiki to family, friends and the people closest to you when they have a need. It is a good idea to allow people to ask you for a treatment rather than simply offering it. You may find yourself in a social situation where someone outside your immediate circle could really benefit from a Reiki treatment. Whilst it may be appropriate for you to tell them about Reiki and explain that this is something you do, it is more appropriate to let them ask you for a treatment. When a person asks, it allows them to create a vortex that Reiki can be received into. If one simply gives, often the person doesn't really receive, because it isn't the right time for them. Perhaps they aren't ready to alter their experience, because their illness or lack of finance is serving a purpose at some personal level. If they do not ask, they haven't opened to the experience, so it is preferable to allow the person to request Reiki themselves.

Reiki stimulates the body's own healing mechanism. Body purification through improved nutrition is advised to enhance the healing process. Talking with the client before the treatment and again afterwards is most helpful and beneficial. It is best to remain quiet during the treatment to encourage releasing and healing to occur. Sometimes a healing crisis may arise during a treatment and it is as well to be prepared for this and have a box of paper tissues in the room, in case of tears during treatment.

What symptoms mean

The body is said to mirror our emotional state, and sometimes stress-related symptoms can be successfully relieved once we become aware of their cause. Events in themselves are never stressful. It is only our reaction that causes us to experience stress. Often we are not aware of the cause on a conscious level. Experiencing a Reiki treatment can be the catalyst for increased awareness and emotional release.

An ache or a pain in itself never happens without cause. Every organ and cell in our bodies is directly or indirectly connected with all the others. If there is discomfort in one area, there are probably several other areas not working sufficiently well to eliminate the problem. Reiki helps to restore harmony as the body is treated holistically.

Sometimes the location of the discomfort can indicate the possible cause. If we are unwilling to acknowledge our feelings at a conscious level, then our body will often do this for us. A student who came for treatment was determined to assure us how happy he was with his chosen subjects. He had become too weak, however, to continue his studies and his parents were anxious he would not achieve the required grades for university entrance. During treatment, however, it became apparent that he was unhappy with his choices and had only taken them to please his parents. Once this was understood, he decided to change course entirely and subsequently he recovered his full health.

A family man was suffering from severe shoulder pain. He had tried all kinds of treatment without success. Whilst talking about his life, it became apparent that he was 'shouldering' too much responsibility. He had literally internalised these feelings, which had surfaced as shoulder pain. Following the Reiki treatment, he decided to make major changes in his life to enable him to delegate his heavy workload and enjoy some of his other interests.

Sometimes the causes of ill-health are more obvious: poor diet, lack of exercise, too much alcohol, smoking and lack of sleep all need to be addressed before the body can function efficiently.

When Reiki is not appropriate

Reiki should not be given after a pre-operative anaesthetic has been administered or during an operation. Reiki increases awareness and would not be helpful in this instance. It creates a balance and harmony in each person's system by reducing toxic residues, which in these circumstances would not be appropriate or desirable. However, Reiki is excellent when used to speed up the healing process after surgery, and it is effective both during and after chemotherapy and radiotherapy. In the earlier edition of this book, it was suggested that the energy would reduce the effectiveness of these treatments. However, since that time it has been shown that this has not been the case and we recommend it highly throughout treatment.

A brief session of 5–10 minutes will be beneficial to anyone (with the exception of anaesthetised pre-operative situations), but individuals taking anti-coagulants or cardiac stimulants should not receive longer than this on a regular basis. This also applies to persons prone to epileptic seizures who are taking medication for this condition. The only exception to this is just before or just after a seizure.

Should there be any reason to assume that an individual has a serious mental or physical disorder of any kind, which you are not qualified to deal with, then it is suggested that you refer the client immediately to a suitably qualified person. If a client is taking medication and you are unsure whether Reiki will complement their treatment, ask their medical practitioner or alternatively advise the person concerned to ask their doctor whether it would be appropriate.

Reiki can be helpful in overcoming alcohol or drug addiction as it promotes deeper levels of awareness. It is always inadvisable to treat a client under the influence of alcohol or drugs. It is important to advise any client to drink more water before and after treatment and ideally to avoid alcohol for at least twenty-four hours following treatment.

Some Reiki Masters recommend that Reiki should not be given to a person wearing a pacemaker or other such aids. It would be wise to err on the side of caution, and if first aid is to be given to a person with such a device, to only treat the areas further away from it.

For the most part, with the exception of the above, there are few instances in which it would not be appropriate to give Reiki. Trust your instincts, and if it feels right to give a treatment, then it is likely to be beneficial.

When Reiki doesn't seem to work

One of the things that Reiki teaches you is tremendous detachment. You become a channel for the energy, allowing the energy to flow through you as you make it available for other people. It is appropriate that you allow the other person to do with the energy whatever they choose, without being attached to the outcome. That is why it is important to allow someone else to ask you for a Reiki treatment, rather than just offer it. Those who come for a treatment because they have been persuaded to, or have come along to prove that something like Reiki couldn't possibly work, will to some extent block the effectiveness of the Reiki energy, because of their own resistance.

The results of Reiki treatments are unpredictable and expectations may not be promptly fulfilled. As Reiki channels we are merely observers, and it is important we do not become judgemental should the desired outcome not be achieved.

Sometimes the person may lose too many secondary benefits if his or her symptoms are removed. However much the individual may assure you they wish to get well, they may also be receiving an exceptional amount of attention from their families whilst unwell, which they might be unwilling to give up should their symptoms be removed. At an unconscious level, they may be resisting the healing process.

One such person who came for healing had forged a marvellous relationship with his previously distant father whilst confined to a wheelchair with post-viral fatigue syndrome. It was clear he was unwilling to risk losing this warm relationship by being able to regain the use of his legs, and he soon stopped treatment.

Another person during an illness was able to adopt a strong role within the hierarchy of her family that she was reluctant to relinquish. No method of healing would have succeeded during this time. At an unconscious level she was choosing illness rather than health.

Some individuals have strong opinions which would prevent them benefiting from a remedy which falls outside their accepted belief system. It is important they are able to freely choose their own method of healing. Reiki simply may not be right for them and they may not believe that such an ethereal form of treatment could remove their symptoms. This is their right, and Reiki is simply not a suitable form of treatment for some people.

These examples are unusual. It is, however, helpful to be aware of the possibility of such situations occurring. The majority of situations provide marvellous and often unexplained opportunities for growth and fulfilment for both the person being treated and the healer.

Group treatments

Reiki works well as a group treatment and is most nurturing for the person receiving the treatment. It is possible for two, three, four or even five people to take part in a group session. The energy is amplified with more people channelling the energy. After Reiki First Degree training, it is helpful to attend group sessions especially for initiates, sometimes known as sharing groups or energy exchanges. These group sessions are an ideal time to get together for an enjoyable healing evening and are far less formal than a one-to-one session.

Everybody is grouped around the table and each person takes it in turn to receive the energy. One person lies on the treatment couch and the others move around the different positions. The person who sits behind the head usually keeps time, if there is not a timed music CD playing. Each person remains in one position for three to five minutes and then moves to the next position until the group has completed that individual's treatment. It is then the turn of the next member of the group to be treated, and so on, until all have given and received in this manner.

This is an excellent way for a novice healer to develop kinaesthetic ability and gain experience in a group setting. It is a good opportunity to share experiences and ask any questions that arise.

ENERGY CIRCLE

An energy exchange usually begins with an energy circle. This allows the group to form an energetic circuit or link by joining hands for a moment or two and letting the energy flow around the circle. The energy circle exercise can be successfully extended into a meditation as well.

GROUP MEDITATION

During this session, a group meditation is usually shared and distant healing is sent to people and situations. Group healing sent to war-torn areas or to friends in hospital is more powerful than when it is sent individually. Any excess of energy is then used to heal the earth.

Sending Reiki through time and space

Reiki can be sent without a person being present using the method taught at Second Degree level. Usually a list of where and to whom the energy is to be sent is compiled by the group at the start of the evening. Before the group distant healing session, one member may read the list out aloud. The group sitting in a circle is then asked to visualise a ball of healing energy in the centre. Those not using the Reiki Second Degree method of distant healing could imagine their hands positioned over the ball of energy channelling more Reiki into the centre of the ball, which then grows larger and larger, until it is sent out to benefit all the people and situations throughout the world on the list previously read out.

As each sharing group collectively sends energy to world situations, the energy becomes amplified many times. The healing that results directly affects us all. There are numerous possibilities for sending Reiki to health or environmental crises worldwide.

Miracles happen every day. Now some people don't think so. But they do.

FORREST GUMP

CHAPTER ELEVEN

Combining Reiki with Other Healing Arts

REIKI COMBINES WELL WITH OTHER complementary therapies, and indeed with conventional forms of medicine. Increasingly more doctors, healing practitioners, masseurs, physical therapists and psychologists participate in Reiki training workshops and combine Reiki with other forms of treatment. The possibilities for combining the various techniques are endless.

Reiki and aromatherapy, reflexology, shiatsu, massage and other bodywork

Those who practise reflexology, massage, aromatherapy, shiatsu and other forms of bodywork find their work is enhanced by combining it with Reiki.

Whether or not Reiki is used formally in conjunction with a particular type of bodywork, the healing energy is transmitted whenever a treatment is given. One massage therapist did not tell her clients she had taken Reiki training and didn't intentionally use it in combination with the massage treatment. The following week a particularly sensitive person who came for a regular massage asked why the treatment that day had felt special, even though the therapist had not done anything different.

Some therapists like to keep treatments separate and offer

perhaps a Reiki treatment one week and their particular bodywork the next. Others prefer to use them in combination. The variations are infinite.

Additionally, aromatherapy and other massage oils can be charged with Reiki by holding the container in cupped hands to be treated for a few moments before the massage. The effectiveness and potency of the ingredients are enhanced. The energy passes easily through glass and plastic, as well as through plaster casts and of course clothes; in fact through anything.

Burning essential oils (usually a few drops diluted into water) whilst giving a Reiki treatment is powerfully therapeutic. Recommended oils include lavender, which promotes relaxation; clary sage, which is known to be a powerful stimulant to awaken the third eye; sandalwood, which has a nurturing quality to promote relaxation; and lemon verbena, which assists in the releasing of old ideas and patterns of behaviour.

Reiki and meditation

Whilst being attuned, participants in Reiki workshops find they naturally slip into a meditative state, even if they have never meditated before. Those who do meditate on a regular basis find that their meditation deepens considerably after being attuned and they are able to achieve a deeper state for longer periods more effortlessly. See Chapter Fifteen for further details on meditation.

Reiki and medicine

Reiki also combines well with conventional medicine. Doctors who have taken Reiki training can use Reiki to diminish pain and reduce anxiety whilst in the process of setting bones, or to speed up healing of post-operative scars. Paediatricians find it helpful in the treatment of young patients. New-born babies in intensive care benefit from Reiki treatment. Many nurses are drawn to Reiki and can use it effectively to soothe patients' suffering, relieve pain and accelerate the healing process. Doctors who have taken Second Degree Reiki have sent their patients distant healing during consultations, which has subsequently assisted the healing process.

Reiki can also reduce the toxic effect of medicines and drugs. The side effects are minimised. Additionally using Reiki may mean that less medication is required for pain relief in a post-operative situation. The possibilities are endless.

Reiki and homeopathy

Reiki works well in conjunction with homeopathic treatments. The remedies can be treated with Reiki before being taken, making them more effective.

Reiki and flower remedies

Flower remedies are the life force essence of flowers. They are a vibrational medicine and work in a similar way to homeopathic remedies. They help to activate the body's own self-healing mechanism by raising the vibrational level of energy patterns. Flower remedies work well in conjunction with Reiki.

Reiki and the chakras

Many forms of energy medicine recognise the existence of a number of energy points known as chakras in different locations over the body. Originating in India, chakras have been described as energy centres. There are seven main chakra points, which clairvoyants see as rotating wheels or spiralling discs of light. Each chakra is said to vibrate at a different rate through being charged by the energy of the sun entering them in the form of light. This causes each chakra to resonate with a particular vibrational frequency. Crystals, flower essences and homeopathic medicines each have vibrational frequencies that the chakras respond to, which evoke a healing response by means of sympathetic resonance.

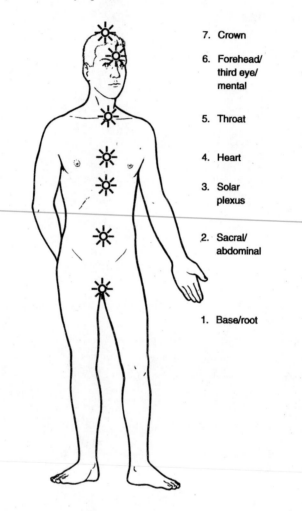

7. Crown

6. Forehead/ third eye/ mental

5. Throat

4. Heart

3. Solar plexus

2. Sacral/ abdominal

1. Base/root

The etheric body, which envelops the physical body, absorbs fine levels of energy and information from the environment through the chakra points. The positions of the chakra points correspond to the endocrine glands in the physical body. The endocrine system controls the hormone balance within a person. The hormones have a powerful effect on the moods and emotions of the individual. If the chakras are out of balance, then it often happens that the endocrine system is also out of sorts and the person concerned may be suffering as a result.

It is no coincidence that the Reiki hand positions are also over the main chakra points. Sometimes it may happen that one particular chakra is not working too well. When this happens, all the chakras fall out of balance. It is far better to treat all the chakras to restore balance throughout the body. This is why a full Reiki treatment is preferable to shorter sessions.

As a human being matures, the chakras also develop and mature. If a person's development is inhibited for any reason, their functioning may be reduced, which could affect their state of health. Reiki treatments restore and balance a person's chakras, enhancing well-being at all levels.

The seven major chakra positions are as follows:

THE BASE CHAKRA

This is in the lower pelvic area and governs the reproductive area, the spinal column and the kidneys. It is in this area that our will for survival is at its most powerful. Unless this chakra is functioning properly, a person cannot develop harmoniously. Blockages may result in mental symptoms, rigid attitudes to life and extreme opinions. On a physical level, a malfunctioning base chakra can result in physical symptoms of the bones, teeth and spine as well as degenerative illnesses and complaints of the large intestine, the ovaries, bladder, uterus and prostate. The corresponding colour is red.

THE SACRAL CHAKRA

This is in the lower abdominal region and governs our ability to perceive the world and interact with it. This is the area of our self-perception and our sexual expression. Blockages in this area can result in fear of physical closeness, frigidity, impotence and diseases relating to our body fluids or the organs processing these fluids, such as the kidneys, lymph glands and bladder. The colour for this chakra is orange.

THE SOLAR PLEXUS CHAKRA

This is situated between the abdomen and the breast-bone and is the area from which we draw our personal power. The solar plexus chakra governs the left side of the brain and is associated with the intellect. It is linked to the pancreas, gall bladder and digestive processes. Blockages result in mental symptoms, changes in personal status and false claims to power. Physical symptoms include stomach and pancreatic complaints as well as digestive disorders. Disorders can produce excessively dominant behaviour. The colour for this chakra is yellow.

THE HEART CHAKRA

This is over the heart and is our emotional centre. This area governs our relationship issues and if balanced allows us to accept the world and other people as they are. It is also the area of self-love. Blockages in this area result in mental symptoms, such as inflexibility and often manipulation in relationships with others, with a reduced capacity to give and receive love. Physical symptoms frequently result in conditions such as heart complaints and malfunctioning of the thymus gland, as well as circulatory disorders, lung diseases, cramps and spasms. Emotional blockages can result in depression or particularly self-sacrificing behaviour. The colour for this chakra is green.

THE THROAT CHAKRA

This chakra is situated over the throat and governs the area of self-expression. This area also regulates metabolism and is associated with communication. Blockages can result in extremely dominant behaviour. Chakra imbalance in this area can sometimes be diagnosed through irregular voice pitch and tone. Physical symptoms can include general disturbances to growth and development, and disorders of the tonsils and throat. There is a connection between the throat and the solar plexus chakras. Imbalance of this chakra can result in tendencies to exert excessive power over others. The colour for this chakra is turquoise blue.

THE THIRD EYE CHAKRA

This is situated in the centre of the forehead and governs our intuition. On a physical level, this chakra affects the pituitary and pineal glands, which influence growth. This area corresponds to the creative right side of the brain and is associated with our inner vision. People whose third eye chakra functions particularly well often develop clairvoyance. Blockages can result in headaches, visual problems, hyperactivity and, conversely, sluggishness.

Hyperactivity of this chakra can result in excessive mental activity. This can lead to a multitude of 'visions'. These 'visions' can often be of an alarming and possibly threatening nature. This may also be accompanied by increased fear and reduced clarity.

Under-functioning of this chakra may cause lack of interest in the world, aimlessness, and absence of personal vision, with a tendency to feel disconnected. The colour for this chakra is indigo.

THE CROWN CHAKRA

This chakra is situated on the top of the head and is linked to the pineal gland. This is our spiritual centre, and from here we develop and interpret our understanding of love, beauty, art and religion, and our connection to all living things and to the divine. Blockages can result in feelings of isolation, seclusion and despair. A crown chakra that is functioning well enables the individual to develop a greater understanding as to the nature of the divine. The colour for this chakra is purple.

CHAKRA BALANCING

To assess the condition of the chakra system, it is possible to use your hands to sense where the movement has slowed down. A clairvoyant may see whether the wheels of light are spinning appropriately. Should there not be enough time for a full Reiki treatment, the chakras can be balanced during a short session.

USING REIKI TO BALANCE THE CHAKRAS

With the person to be treated sitting in a chair, place one hand on the forehead and one on the back of the neck. Then place both hands on the shoulders. After this, place one hand on the chest and one on the back. Next, place one hand on the solar plexus and one hand on the corresponding position on the back. Finally, place one hand on the abdomen and one hand on the tailbone. This short treatment will balance the chakras effectively.

CHAKRA BALANCING EXERCISE

Make yourself comfortable sitting upright on a chair and take two or three deep breaths.

Allow your breath to become regular, and as you breathe in again, breathe in the colour red. See your entire body fill with the colour. Slowly bring your awareness to your pelvic region. Visualise a spiral of red light spinning (looking directly at the chakra from outside the body) under your body in the pelvic region.

When this spiral of red light is spinning vigorously, visualise yourself breathing in orange, filling yourself with orange light. See a spiral of orange light spinning in the abdomen region.

Following this, feel yourself breathing in yellow. Visualise your entire being filling with yellow light as you breathe in and out. Bring your attention to the solar plexus region. See a spiral of yellow light spinning there.

Next, allow yourself to breathe in green. With each breath, breathe in more green light. Focus on your heart chakra and visualise a green spiral spinning powerfully with every breath that you take.

And now see yourself breathing in blue. Feel yourself filling up with blue light. Focus on your throat area and visualise a blue spinning spiral rotating in your throat area as you breathe in the blue light.

Next, breathe in indigo, the combined colour of blue and violet. Visualise this colour filling your body as you breathe in and out. Focus on your third eye area, feel the indigo spinning spiral moving into the third eye with every breath.

Next, breathe in violet. See your whole body filling up with violet light. Concentrate your focus on the crown area on the top of your head. See a spiral of violet light spinning in this area. Feel it with every breath taken in.

Now, breathe in pure white light. Fill yourself with bright white light. See the spiral of white light begin to spin powerfully on to and around the top of your head, spreading throughout your entire body. See this column of brilliant white light cascading down, purifying, invigorating and energising your whole system, which is now connected to this vast column of white light, stretching up to infinity.

When you are ready, and your chakras are sufficiently charged, take a few deep breaths and then slowly open your eyes.

Clearing energy blockages

Energy flows freely through the body when we are in optimum health physically, emotionally and mentally. When we feel threatened or view the world as an unsafe place, we create energy blocks, which reduce the flow of energy through our systems.

Occasionally whilst giving treatments, certain areas may seem to draw less energy than the surrounding areas, and may even feel cool to the touch. You may intuitively sense that an energy block is present. Reiki is very powerful and will gently break down such blocks, given time. To speed the breakdown of such a blockage, visualise yourself grasping the stuck energy and pulling it up and out of the system. See yourself severing its connection to the body with your hand and either project a laser beam from your third eye area to dissipate it or pass it on to angels or beings of light, who remove it. This exercise will free the area concerned and you may well find that area now accepting more Reiki energy than previously. For more information on types of energy blocks and dispersing them, read *Hands of Light* by Barbara Brennan.

Sound and Reiki

Sound has a powerful therapeutic effect. Singing and chanting have always profoundly affected mood and well-being. The powerful vibrational frequency of sound has the potential to be used for healing far more extensively than at present. Tribal people have always used singing and chanting to connect with their environment, entertain, lift their spirits and heal their sick.

Musician Steve Halpern, amongst others, composes music relating to specific sound frequencies in order to stimulate healing. His compositions have been played in numerous clinics and hospitals, achieving successful responses from a great many people. The resonance of this music is said to tune the chakra system and enhance well-being.

Many voice and sound workshops teach various types of singing and chanting. They have enabled people to re-connect with the power of their own voice and use it for healing and enjoyment. The singing these groups are guided to produce in such workshops is astonishingly beautiful and never fails to surprise and delight the participants. Not so long ago, Western scientists identified a particular resonance as having properties that evoked a powerful healing response. This resonance was apparently identical to that emitted by the gong, which has been used for healing by traditional cultures for centuries.

Music is often played in the background whilst a Reiki treatment is being given. Almost any tranquil music is appropriate. There are now a great many choices available, including some specially composed for Reiki treatments. The Internet is a good place to search for a variety of suitable music.

Colour and Reiki

All the colours of the rainbow are used in healing, and each one has its own effect. There are many books available on colour's powerful healing effects. Each one of us uses colour therapy when we select a particular colour to wear each day. Hospitals have been known to use particular colours on their walls to speed up healing responses. Prisons have experimented with colours to reduce aggression. Colour therapy, or chromatherapy, is often used at holistic spas and health centres for therapeutic effect. It is rooted in Ayurveda, an ancient form of medicine practised in India for thousands of years, and was used in ancient Egypt and China. When a particular colour is absent from the auric field of the individual, ill health often results. A specially trained therapist can determine which colour is most needed and the person is enveloped in colour rays from specially designed lights.

Colourpuncture is a fusion of traditional Chinese medicine and colour therapy. It involves focusing coloured lights on acupuncture and other points on the body to initiate powerful healing impulses. The cells of the body communicate with each other through the medium of light and each colour communicates different energetic information. Like Reiki, colourpuncture addresses the emotional origin of illnesses as well as the physical symptoms. Further information can be found at www.colourpuncture.com

A Reiki practitioner may visualise a particular colour being beamed to a person during a treatment. Sometimes it is helpful to advise a client to wear more of a particular colour. An under-active chakra, for example, can be restored by being stimulated with the appropriate colour.

There is always a long line of people waiting at Mind Body & Spirit type exhibitions to have a photograph of their aura taken and then interpreted. At one such exhibition, an exhibitor was displaying photographs of a person's aura before and after a Reiki treatment. There was a multitude of colours in the auric field following the treatment.

Some healers with clairvoyant ability are able to detect illness in the auric field before it manifests in the physical body.

The following exercise can be used in the shower, or simply as a meditation to relax and restore you at any time, in which case a waterfall may be substituted as a more appropriate setting.

TAKING A COLOUR SHOWER

Imagine as you take a shower that the water has a magical quality, being able to radiate each of the brilliant colours of the rainbow.

As you switch on the shower and step into it, visualise the vibrant red colour of the water warming and energising you. As this colour pours down on you, take a moment to feel yourself infused with the beautiful, vibrant red colour, releasing all your fears.

Then see the water become a brilliant shade of orange. Orange opens you to experience joy and allows you to release shame and guilt. Orange relieves cramp and strengthens the bronchial tubes. Feel the orange colour around you.

Now see the water becoming a bright shade of yellow. Feel the yellow water cleanse emotional pain and stimulate the lymphatic system. Yellow clears the mind and invigorates the digestion.

Visualise the water becoming a brilliant shade of green, balancing and restoring the physical body and stimulating the pituitary gland. Green purifies the whole system, renewing your expression of love and forgiveness.

See the water change to a beautiful, cooling, magical blue. Blue enhances self-expression, allowing you to speak your truth. Feel the blue all around you, allowing you to express yourself according to your true self.

The water changes to indigo and purple. Visualise yourself surrounded by indigo and purple, stimulating your own healing power and wisdom. Indigo stimulates the third eye, awakening your intuition, and purple increases your cosmic connection. Feel the calming influence of the velvet dark colours of indigo and purple.

Finally, visualise the water becoming brilliant white light. White takes away any pain and shows you the peace and joy within your own spirit. Take a moment to enjoy the white light surrounding you, filling you with peace and harmony, before finishing your rainbow shower.

Crystals and Reiki

A powerful resonance exists between living beings and crystals. Crystals can be used with Reiki to promote healing in many ways. Crystals are said to amplify and focus energy that can be directed at specific energy blockages in order to repair disruptive patterns in the etheric field, sometimes even before a physical illness has manifested. They cannot, however, remove the negative thought patterns that may have contributed to causing the illness in the first place. This is where Reiki can help by its effect at a causal level. Crystals can work well in conjunction with Reiki.

QUARTZ CRYSTALS FOR ENERGY BLOCKS

Quartz crystals are especially effective for powerfully directing healing energy and breaking down blockages. They are a helpful supplement to Reiki healing, being ideal for programming with healing thought forms. They can treat specific organs and disorders as well as having a calming effect on people who normally find it difficult to relax.

Quartz crystals can be used as a way of removing an energy block during a Reiki treatment. It is best to use a long crystal for this purpose. When an area appears to be drawing very little or no energy, point the crystal at the block and move it rapidly in a clockwise direction, up and away, to free up the blockage. This area may then receive more energy.

Quartz can be used in a similar manner to repair damaged chakras or energise scar tissue. Crystals can be placed in a particular position on the person receiving a Reiki treatment to further help a particular organ or to generally complement the energy.

Quartz crystals radiate much beauty and light and can be carried easily in the pocket to heighten positive interaction with others on a daily basis. In a working environment where there is a certain amount of ongoing conflict, it is often recommended that quartz crystals are regularly cleansed and re-programmed for effective results.

AMETHYST CRYSTALS AND INTUITIVE DEVELOPMENT

Amethyst reflects the purple ray, which is one of the colours for the third eye centre and symbolises change of consciousness and altered awareness. It is, therefore, most effective for stimulating the awakening of the third eye and intuitive abilities. It helps to raise general awareness and encourages self-development. Amethyst also brings clarity to allow us to recognise our own individual path, and conveys vitality so that we are able to follow it. Amethyst is ideal to use when meditating. It can also be placed directly on the third eye to stimulate it, and can usher in a tranquil state of inner calm. It works well in conjunction with rose quartz, which soothes and opens the heart, to bring about a peaceful balance of mental and emotional energies.

ROSE QUARTZ FOR HEALING TRAUMA

Rose quartz opens the heart as its warm pink vibration corresponds directly to the heart chakra. It can heal trauma and release deep blockages as well as feelings of anxiety. The properties of this crystal heal deep wounds and allow you to open to self-love and the love of others. It is a stone for those who have never before been able to experience the joy of living. Often when children are brought up without the love and nurturing they need, they are unable to love themselves and subsequently cannot love others. Unless deep inner healing takes place, that person is trapped in a vicious circle, unable to provide love for their own children. Rose quartz allows healing to take place by penetrating the inner chamber of the heart chakra and dissolving the emotional burdens trapped within. Rose quartz would be an ideal complement to Reiki when healing heart issues, as the stone could be carried on the person whilst healing continues.

MOONSTONE FOR BALANCING THE EMOTIONS

Moonstone helps to soothe and balance the emotions and acts as a guardian at the gateway to the subconscious. This allows a greater awareness to unfold. Moonstone is very good for balancing the masculine and feminine aspects of ourselves. It helps men to become more in tune with the feminine side of themselves and allows women greater emotional and hormonal balance during their menstrual cycle. Moonstones help to neutralise negative emotions, allowing calmness and peace of mind to prevail.

Many books and courses are now available on the subject of crystals, and there are numerous possibilities for combining Reiki with every different type of crystal for healing and transformation.

Reiki, imagery and healing

Images are common in Reiki and can sometimes offer clues as to the origin of an illness. Imagery is a powerful medium, and it is sometimes possible to use the images received in a creative way to elicit a healing response. By altering the images in the mind, a healing response can be initiated. This is a particularly effective technique to use with children.

One child who had a bed-wetting problem received an image of a hosepipe that was out of control. When she was asked to visualise a tap being put in, to control the water and subsequently turn it off, the bed-wetting stopped.

Visualisations are an effective way for the mind to communicate with the body. An appropriately chosen image can produce successful results in numerous situations. The only difficulty is determining the most appropriate image. This can only be done by the person who is unwell. It is possible to help someone find such an image, though it would be impossible to compile an ideal list of visualisations for illnesses, as the image needs to be personalised and adapted for individual use (see Further Reading, page 168).

When Reiki is being sent to you for a specific problem, observe any images that come to mind. Often people who, for example, have inflammation in a particular area visualise a fire. In that instance, it may be appropriate to visualise the flames being put out, plus steps to ensure the fire can never start again. It is more effective with your own image and it lets you take an active part in your healing process.

Reiki and arts therapies

Art, dance and music therapies help people to express emotion and thoughts they would otherwise find hard to articulate. There are times when Reiki makes you aware of some deeply repressed emotion or a situation you feel uncomfortable with. Being able to draw how you feel, or act it out, can help you communicate more easily. Reiki combines well with all arts therapies.

CHAPTER TWELVE

Diet, Exercise and Reiki

A healthy body

IN THE UK ALONE, obesity has trebled since 1980 and heart disease is the number one killer. Reiki can help you to stay healthy by boosting your immune system so you resist infections, but eating the right food, keeping your weight under control and staying active is up to you.

KEEPING FIT

We are all familiar with the notion that exercise is good for us, but if we aren't ill, why exercise at all? Quite apart from staving off obesity and the subsequently related illnesses, we exercise because it keeps our hearts and lungs in good condition, as well as stretching and toning the muscles. It also encourages the body to release endorphins, the chemicals which enhance mood and add a feel-good factor to our lives.

FROM FAT TO FINN

Take a tip from the Finns, who have dramatically changed their diet and lifestyle; from having the world's highest rate of heart disease, they are now one of the healthiest nations on earth. This spectacular turnaround began in 1972, when the people of North Karelia asked for government help for the area's exceptionally high level of coronary heart disease. The response was a project that was so successful it was adopted with enthusiasm by the rest of the country. Their desire to change led to the ideas snowballing and spreading to every walk of life. This included schools, universities and the workplace, as well as the home. The results were outstanding. Just five years after the programme began, deaths from heart disease in men under 65 had fallen by 82 per cent. Life expectancy for both sexes rose by ten years. Regular exercise has become a way of life for 70 per cent of the Finnish people.

Here are some tips from the Finnish project:

1. Cut out packaged food with low nutritional value and high fat and sugar content.
2. Eat lots of green vegetables and fresh fruit.
3. Choose low-fat options wherever possible.
4. Use vegetable oils instead of fatty milk products.
5. Use less high-fat dairy produce, choosing low-fat options instead.
6. Choose lean meat and plenty of fish.
7. Make exercise a regular part of your life.
8. Supplement your diet, if only with a good-quality multi-vitamin daily.
9. Change your focus to health, not sickness.

Syndrome X

A condition known as Syndrome X (or metabolic syndrome) is rapidly gaining recognition in the medical world. It was unheard of just a decade ago, yet is becoming increasingly common. The condition is characterised by a number of biochemical and bodily imbalances that include weight gain (typically around the stomach area), raised cholesterol levels and high blood pressure. It is believed to affect around a quarter of adults in the UK. If affected, there is a strong possibility that a person will go on to develop type II diabetes and heart disease.

The cause of Syndrome X is unknown, but theorists believe that a sedentary lifestyle is an important factor in the growing rates of obesity, as is a diet laden with sugar and processed carbohydrates (white flour, white rice, pasta and most cakes, pastries and biscuits).

The good news is that Syndrome X is reversible. Evidence suggests that lower-carbohydrate diets tend to improve the action of insulin. Cutting out sugar-laden foods such as chocolate, cakes and soft drinks and basing your diet on green vegetables, fish, meat, eggs, plenty of salads, fresh fruits, nuts and seeds will be effective in helping you to lose weight and combating Syndrome X.

Daily exercise can also play an important role. The right exercise is the one you enjoy doing. If you can't face exercise, here's a way to get you started. Walk for thirty minutes a day; ten minutes in the morning, ten at lunch and ten in the evening. Take every opportunity to become more active. If the journey isn't far, walk. Use the commercial breaks on television to do some household chores. Walk around when you talk on the telephone or exercise on the spot.

Reiki in conjunction with diet and exercise can help to combat Syndrome X by bringing balance to blood sugar levels and reducing raised blood pressure. At the end of the day, relax in a hot bath, followed by a Reiki treatment. If time is short, treat the heart and liver area; otherwise a full body treatment is recommended.

For further information on Syndrome X, see the section on Further Reading plus the Useful Websites at the back of the book.

Reiki and the food you eat

To get the most out of Reiki, choose a nutritious diet that will allow your system to gain maximum benefit. This is particularly important following initiation. Forget fast food and ready meals. Use wholesome ingredients and make each meal, however simple, a sacred space to enrich your soul. Choose fresh fruit, vegetables and raw salads, organic wherever possible, lean meat and fish, wholegrain bread, brown rice, oats, barley, buckwheat, bulgar wheat, yoghurt, eggs, nuts, dried fruit and seeds.

Reiki can help to energise your meals.

ENERGISING YOUR FOOD

1. Sit or stand in a comfortable position. Become aware of your breathing. Allow yourself to relax. Breathe more deeply.
2. Visualise Reiki coming through your head, down to your shoulders, through your arms and out of your hands.
3. Think of the people you love, a special moment in your life or anything that evokes loving, caring feelings.
4. Now visualise that the light coming out of your hands is infused with this love. It is shimmering and glowing.
5. Project it on to the food and drink before you and see it soaking into it. Surround both sides of the dish with your hands and feel it emanating from your fingers, infusing the food with a loving, healing energy.

There is far more to food than calories. Take a moment to think about where the food you eat comes from. See orange groves glistening in the sunshine, rows of corn, fields of wheat, lambs or cows grazing. Food contains subtle energies that enrich us. Imagining it in its original surroundings encourages us to obtain the best possible ingredients. All too often, we don't consider the origins of our food. When we do, our eating habits start to change.

Tips to avoid over-eating

Merchandising and food packaging often mean that we are faced with extra-large portion sizes, encouraging over-eating, even though the food is more than our bodies want or need. Food companies often exert subtle and not so subtle influence over our will-power, making it difficult to refuse. Here are some tips to overcome it.

1. Avoid all-you-can-eat buffet-style restaurants or those with particularly large portion sizes. Keep away from fast-food establishments offering inexpensive lunchtime menus with super-size portions. If you find you have to eat in a restaurant with excessive portion sizes, under-estimate when you are ordering or choose to split the main course with someone else.

2. Never choose jumbo-sized popcorn tubs or fizzy drinks at cinemas where you can return for limitless top-ups.

3. When entertaining, try not to offer a range of desserts, as it is too tempting to try a little of each. If you must serve more than one dessert, choose a fruit salad or fresh fruit platter as the second choice.

4. Keep all snacks out of sight, reducing temptation. If you must keep something within reach, ensure it is a healthy snack, such as nuts, seeds, vegetable crudités or fruit.

5. Resist the temptation to buy multi packs of chocolate bars in supermarkets because they are a bargain.

6. Try not to shop when you are hungry, so that you are not tempted to buy calorie-laden snacks.

7. Plan to take healthy snacks to work with you rather than finding yourself in a convenience store with high-fat, sugary alternatives.

Detoxify with Reiki

Have a day to detoxify once a month. Spend twenty-four hours eating only home-made vegetable broths plus raw fruit and vegetable juices. Reiki will assist the process and take away any discomfort from the odd headache you experience as your system starts to detoxify. Your whole system will benefit and you'll feel energised and vibrant.

Find the right diet for you

Choosing the right diet can be bewildering. A highly beneficial way of eating for many people is according to blood group. It is based on the theory that your blood type determines which foods can help you to lose weight and enjoy better health and which you need to avoid. When you eat foods compatible with your blood type, aches, pains and food intolerances disappear. To find out more about the considerable benefits of such a diet, read *Eat Right For Your Type* by Peter D'Adamo. Another weight-loss/energy programme involves testing individual reactions to common foods, so diet can be adapted to suit the individual. One version of this is called Novo by Immogenics. More information and website details can be found at the back of the book.

Enjoy more energy

Sometimes we have all the energy we need, whilst at other times it is sadly lacking. Reiki is a wonderful tool to boost flagging resources when your energy banks are low, but what else can you do to enjoy an abundance of energy whenever you need it?

Invisible, intangible energy is affected by everything in your life: your thoughts, your choice of friends, your colleagues, family members, and how much fun you are having at the time. Having lists of incomplete jobs drains your energy. Worrying and any kind of anxiety rapidly deplete your reserves. Conversely, some people and places make you feel energised, enthusiastic and positive. The trick is to identify the people who regularly drain your energy and distance yourself from them as much as possible. Choose to spend more time with those whose company you enjoy and who understand and inspire you.

We have identified ten steps to help you enjoy more energy, whenever you need it.

Ten steps to endless energy

1. Throw out clutter. Keep surfaces empty by regularly clearing piles of paperwork and magazines that build up.

2. Keep your thinking positive. Don't let your thoughts dwell on the down side. This promotes stress.
3. Vary your routine, doing something different each day.
4. Move around as much as possible during the day, especially at work.
5. Make the effort to do something you love. Take time to enjoy yourself. Laughter is a great energy-booster, increasing the number of feel-good endorphins and reducing the stress hormone cortisol.
6. Set goals, so you always have something to work towards. Energise them by putting them in a Reiki box (see Chapter Six) and sending energy to them.
7. Create time and space for yourself to complete tasks by turning off mobiles and responding to emails or messages only at designated times during the day.
8. Don't let anger build up. If someone is angering you, don't let it escalate. Get your feelings out by discussing it with them. If this isn't possible, put a firm limit on the amount of time you will let it bother you, for example twenty-four hours. If there is nothing further you can do, send Reiki to the situation and release it from your thoughts.
9. Avoid stimulants, such as tea or coffee, late at night. Get enough sleep, plenty of nutritious food and regular exercise.
10. Give yourself Reiki for as little as fifteen minutes a day to keep your energy levels high.

Spend as much time as you can outdoors enjoying fresh air. Natural light makes you feel good, whilst artificial light drains you. It also helps to escape the stale indoor atmosphere and breathe fresh air into your lungs. If possible, keep plenty of plants in the room where you work, so your environment is oxygen rich.

If you still have unexplained fatigue, check it out with your doctor in case you have an iron deficiency or some other underlying disorder.

Other Ways of Using Reiki

If you knew who walks beside you at all times on this path that you have chosen, you would never experience fear again.
A COURSE IN MIRACLES, FOUNDATION FOR INNER PEACE
(PENGUIN, 1997)

Asking for unseen help

Mystical thinkers and sages have always told us that we live in an interactive universe. We did not always believe this to be the case. Some years ago, long before we had discovered Reiki, our own lives seemed to be filled with pain and struggle at one particular point. One evening, we came across a chapter in a book that focused on the possibility of other intelligent beings co-existing alongside ourselves in other dimensions. We remember asking the universe out loud for help that night and subsequently forgetting all about it.

Chris's parents passed away unexpectedly within several months of each other. It was not long after this that we found ourselves sitting in a crowded spiritualist church for the first time in our lives. Whilst listening to the medium passing messages to others, I wondered what I was even doing there, when suddenly she turned to address me. Despite any good intentions, scepticism would not have allowed me to draw comfort from vague 'messages' that would have applied to anyone. Besides, the relationship we had enjoyed with Chris's mother was an uneasy one, to say the least.

One of the first things the medium said was 'They know you have asked for help and help is there from many sources.' Our faces must have registered absolute astonishment, as she then went on to identify Chris's mother and describe her character and physical appearance. The medium cannot have begun to imagine our incredulity when she subsequently delivered a very warm and quite unexpected apology for the way in which our relationship had been conducted. Those few moments were transformational.

Although we were never again to return to the spiritualist church, the thought of having received a response from unseen dimensions was extremely exciting. We spent all our spare time over the following months reading all we could on the nature of metaphysics. We attended lectures, enrolled on courses and generally learned as much as possible about the esoteric nature of the universe. We learned to ask for answers and opportunities. Each time, the universe responded. Sometimes the answer came to mind unexpectedly. Sometimes it would 'coincidentally' be included in a magazine article in a waiting room, or we would be seated next to someone on a train who was just the person to help.

We realised that one of the ways in which the universe works is that you have to ask clearly for what you want, rather like placing your order in a restaurant. When we were later to learn Reiki, the teacher emphasised the importance of this. Be care you don't ask for struggle! If you would like to meet a new partner, be specific. One student who had split up from her partner was disappointed that her relationship hadn't succeeded. She told us that she had asked the universe for a pleasant, kind partner and for some reason it hadn't worked out. I asked her why she was unhappy and it turned out her partner was pleasant enough, but his company wasn't as stimulating as she would have liked. She subsequently made a far more detailed list of characteristics she would like her future partner to have and enlisted the universe's help. Ask for help in finding your future partner but leave the details, such as where, when and how you meet this person, to the universe.

When you ask, you open to the possibility and your vibrational frequency changes. Then you can relax and look out for what you have asked for. Of course, you still need to take action as you would normally. Your soul mate may not find you if you never ventured further than your home! By leaving the agenda to the universe, you are allowing for the possibilities of synchronicity and coincidence to assist the process. It is often said that synchronicity is God's way of remaining anonymous.

One woman missed a job interview because of a rail delay and decided to take an earlier train home. On this train she was to meet her future partner, whom she later married. They subsequently lived by the sea in a warmer climate, which was exactly what she had originally desired.

Whilst it is perfectly acceptable to ask for whatever you would like for yourself, it wouldn't be appropriate to ask on anyone else's behalf. That would be interfering. It may be tempting to ask if someone could win the lottery next Tuesday as they have money worries, but it simply may not be in the best interests of that person to suddenly find themselves extremely wealthy. On the contrary, it may create a whole new set of problems for them. The Beatles were not so wrong when they sang 'Money can't buy me love'; they could have added that 'Money can't buy me happiness either'.

At some level, people may be learning from their lack of abundance and need to work it out for themselves. Somebody once said that it was far better to teach a man to fish than to catch the fish for him, and we have to agree with that. In the long term, it is far better to show someone how they can fix their own problems.

Every time you give yourself a Reiki treatment, be sure to ask for what you want and send energy to where it is most needed. Look out for the delivery.

Reiki and pregnancy

Women who are having a baby enjoy Reiki, as it helps to alleviate many of the usual symptoms, such as morning sickness and lower back pain.

The baby also seems to enjoy it, and there is often a lively kick in response to the energy flow. A daily Reiki treatment (or a weekly treatment if this is not possible), especially on the abdominal area, the heart, the solar plexus and the temple, will help the body to handle the changes and the increased demands that pregnancy puts upon it.

After the birth, Reiki can be used effectively to help the baby recover quickly from the trauma of being born, and can also help with any complication that may arise. The energy will be flowing whenever the mother is stroking or holding the child and this will be very soothing and comforting for the baby.

Reiki has been known to assist the fertility process and has helped when a pregnancy ran into difficulties. The unborn child was given Reiki in addition to a doctor's treatment and was later safely born and healthy.

Reiki and children

> I have many flowers,' he said, 'but the children are the most beautiful flowers of all.
>
> OSCAR WILDE, THE SELFISH GIANT

CHILDREN LEARNING REIKI

As a family, we regularly enjoy energy exchanges. It is a special time. Our son was only eight years old when he was attuned, but before this, he often placed his small hands on the feet of his sisters and joined in with the rest of the family.

One day he asked whether he was really channelling the energy along with the rest of us. We told him truthfully that he wasn't. From that point, he asked nearly every day to be 'tuned', as he called it. Eventually we asked him why he wished to be 'tuned' and he replied that he wanted to be able to give Reiki to his pet hamster and help his friends with their cuts and bruises in the playground.

He was too young to join in a workshop, so we decided to attune him each evening for four nights instead of his bedtime story. He experienced the attunements as brilliant lights and accepted this with both simplicity and wonder. Young children can only channel the energy for short periods, and our son was no different. It was marvellous to see him treat his bruises in a matter-of-fact way and soothe away any aches and discomforts.

If children are old enough and are drawn to learning Reiki, they can enjoy the benefits for themselves.

Many children enjoy learning to meditate too. Starting with just five minutes a day, early in the morning, can bring many benefits. If the location has a tranquil atmosphere, the meditation can become a special time that can have a very calming effect and help the child to stay centred throughout the day. It might be the beginning of a lifelong habit and become a source of great peace for the child.

Babies and children really enjoy receiving Reiki and it is useful for first aid when treating minor injuries. Reiki also supports the healing in the case of serious illness, as well as minor problems on a day-to-day basis. It is a most loving, nurturing way of caring for a baby and will intensify the relationship between the mother and the child. From soothing any colic that a baby might experience, to reducing teething discomfort, Reiki can be helpful to ease pain and reduce inflammation. Treatment of babies and children generally does not take long, and a few moments can be enough. Absent healing can help an apprehensive child or soothe a crying baby in another room. As babies grow into children, Reiki is a wonderful way to nurture them.

REIKI AND NIGHTMARES

Reiki can help ease many of childhood's difficult times, especially in conjunction with visualisation. One way of helping a child to regain confidence after experiencing a nightmare would be to comfort the child, and when they are feeling safe and secure, place one hand on their forehead and the other on the solar plexus area and allow the energy to flow. At the same time, it may be helpful to use the following visualisation to assist the child in overcoming the feelings of fear and helplessness that the nightmare has caused.

VISUALISATION FOLLOWING NIGHTMARES

(Adapted from *Creative Visualisations with Children* by Jennifer Day, HarperCollins, 1994)

You are in a very safe place and there is love all around you. Very safe, peaceful and comforting. As you look around you in this very safe, peaceful place, you can see that monster (or whatever the child fears) and because you are in such a safe, peaceful place, you are in control of everything that happens here. As you look at the monster, you feel yourself becoming larger and larger, and as you look at the monster, you can see that it is becoming smaller and smaller, until it is so small, it is small enough to play with. The monster is now so small, it is the size of a toy and you can play with it, roll it around or play a game with it. And if you want it to go away, you can throw it up in the air where it will travel far away to outer space and never return again.

Reiki for first aid

In addition to common sense and first aid procedures, Reiki can be used to help treat a wide range of unexpected injuries. For example, in the event of someone cutting themselves, a bandage can be applied and the whole area treated with Reiki to speed up healing. When a person is in shock, giving them Reiki can help to calm them down and prevent unnecessary trauma from setting in. If bones are broken, it is best not to treat the area of the fracture, but to treat the forehead and the back of the head to soothe the person whilst awaiting help. After the bone has been set, it is then helpful to treat the area directly.

Reiki can help with whiplash injuries in addition to cold compresses applied directly over the affected area. Giving Reiki to the injured area will speed up the healing process. Cuts and bruises benefit greatly from Reiki. If the cut is anything more than minor, and especially when bleeding is excessive, go immediately to the hospital Accident and Emergency unit for treatment.

Reiki can help with minor burns. Where the skin is unbroken, the area can be treated with the sap from the aloe vera plant, if available. If the skin is broken, then a bandage should be applied. Reiki can then treat the burned area without making direct contact. It is also helpful to use visualisation to envisage the whole area being healed. The length and area of treatment depend on the comfort of the person being treated. For anything more than minor burns, seek professional help.

Reiki is effective in treating insect bites, especially in conjunction with homeopathic remedies, such as apis mellifica. Applying one drop of peppermint oil directly on to the bite or sting helps too. Sprains can be helped greatly with Reiki, which sometimes brings relief in a surprisingly short space of time. Treat the area directly wherever possible. Tubular bandages are often helpful too. As a general rule, leave your hands over the area being treated for as long as the person feels comfortable. Learning basic first aid procedures is helpful as well and a useful addition to the skills of any healing practitioner.

Reiki and dreams

It is never advisable to interpret anyone else's dreams. However, you can use Reiki to help yourself or someone else to understand their dreams. We often have dreams that symbolise our current circumstances, and understanding them can clarify our perspective. Often the elements in a dream can represent different aspects of us. We have may facets to our complex personalities and, whilst resting or dreaming, our subconscious mind can re-enact a particular scenario that represents in symbol form the situation that we find ourselves in.

To open the dream, there are three questions that you may ask yourself or another person to begin to gain some clarity as to its meaning.

- How did you feel in the dream (i.e., sad, happy, fearful, distressed, angry, etc.)?
- How would you have liked the dream to end?
- Can you relate the dream to any particular situation in your everyday life?

Before giving yourself a Reiki treatment, you can set the intent either that you will experience that dream again, or, better still, that you will know by the end of the treatment or by the following day its meaning. It is surprising how many times the answer will come to you in this way.

Reiki and de-cluttering your home

The most common reaction to giving oneself a daily Reiki treatment at First Degree level is 'I can never find that sort of time' or 'I simply don't have a spare hour – or a spare five minutes'. It is a sad fact of modern life that even with all kinds of appliances designed to save our time, we find we are busier than ever. Our cupboards overflow with time-saving gadgets, we have devices to enable us to cook faster, wash and dry our clothes, clean our plates, reheat faster, boil faster, help us to lose weight faster, entertain us; yet we still haven't time to enjoy the sunset.

The truth is, we have been so busy amassing all the things we believe we need, in order to enjoy life more and free up our time, that we haven't noticed our lives becoming more fragmented, as we cram as much as we can into each moment. It is no wonder that stress-related disorders are becoming increasingly commonplace.

Practitioners of the Oriental art of feng shui assess how to maximise the flow of energy through your home with the design of the space and the arrangements of the contents. Another aspect of feng shui is space-clearing. This is a procedure which clears a room of stale energy. Space-clearing works well in conjunction with Reiki.

Reiki Second Degree techniques can be used effectively to energetically cleanse a room. The room actually feels better, with technical disturbances being substantially reduced or even completely removed.

Similarly, Reiki can help to dispose of our inner clutter by connecting us to our insight and wisdom. If we can simplify our lives, we can relax more. It is as simple as that. It is up to us to dispose of our outer clutter, so that we have the space for inner tranquillity.

In our homes, we often amass a far greater quantity of items than we are able to use. Our houses are full of clutter: out-of-date magazines, piles of paperwork, half-read books, unwanted gifts lurking at the back of cupboards, redundant kitchen gadgets, old crockery, and toys and games that no one will ever play with again.

So many charities will come and collect household paraphernalia, yet we often hang on to it, sometimes to link us to the past or in case we might need it in the future. If we were to clear it all out, recycle it and just keep what we are using right now, the home would be far simpler to maintain.

A wise man once observed that if we were meant to be so frenetically busy all the time, we would have been called 'human doings'. By simplifying our lives in whatever ways we see fit, we can enjoy far more harmony and inner balance.

Abundance and prosperity programming

The truly rich are those who enjoy what they have.
ANONYMOUS (YIDDISH PROVERB)

Our beliefs often keep us from experiencing the abundance we desire. Money is simply another form of energy and in itself is neither positive nor negative. We can attract to ourselves whatever we require once we explore and break through self-imposed barriers. Money is a thought form. It is a symbol of energy, neither good nor bad. Whereas for some the love of money can cause them to become greedy and corrupt, it is not 'the root of all evil', as it has been depicted. Without money you can't be free, and that is quite a limitation to place upon yourself. Often the difference between success and failure, abundance and poverty is just a small, subtle shift in consciousness.

Money is, of course, only one form of abundance. There is also the abundance of happiness, love, friendship and experience. People lacking money often lack in other areas too. It is important to be open to receive. When extra money is offered, many people turn it down, perhaps believing it is 'not right' to accept. When unexpected money comes your way, choose to accept it. In this way you open yourself to the abundance of the universe. If you see yourself in terms of energy, the work you do or investments you make are a part of that overall energy. Therefore, the money you receive from those efforts is also energy. By seeing money in energetic terms, you can open yourself up to infinite amounts of energy. It is unlimited. Many people have negative conceptions about money and it is this belief that keeps them lacking. Abundance never relates to how much someone has. Rather it is a measure of how a person feels about money. Having said that, money doesn't automatically grant happiness or good health. There are plenty of miserable billionaires to testify to that. It does, however, give you the freedom to buy interesting experiences and help others.

Use your intuition to know when to take a chance on a potential money-making proposition. We are all connected by what Jung termed 'the collective unconscious'. All information is accessible through our inner knowing. Instead of seeing departed relations floating through your hallways, decide to use your intuition to know whether to invest in a potentially lucrative enterprise. Allow yourself to dream the winning lottery number, and don't forget to buy a ticket! Take a chance, you can only be wrong! When you give yourself a Reiki treatment, choose to send energy to your abundance. When the universe responds, accept it. Paula Horan has written an excellent book called *Abundance Through Reiki*, which describes a self-help programme that explores belief patterns and promotes your own natural ability to experience creativity, freedom and abundance.

Increase your confidence with Reiki

All that we are is the result of what we have thought.
The mind is everything. What we think, we become.

BUDDHA

All too often many of us seek approval from others instead of giving ourselves the appreciation we deserve. As a result we often undermine our achievements and never feel completely comfortable with ourselves. This could be due to upbringing or cultural conditioning, which has enforced the belief that thinking a lot of yourself is simply wrong. With confidence and a strong sense of self-worth, you can reach great heights. Without them, even the simplest accomplishments seem out of reach. Confidence comes from within and begins with liking yourself and approving of who you are. It is about believing in yourself when nobody else does.

In the following exercise, recall the five things you most like about yourself.

Five things I like about myself are:

1. _____
2. _____
3. _____
4. _____
5. _____

What is really special about you?

Three things that really mark me out as unique are:

1. _____
2. _____
3. _____

Is there anything else you have missed? Write another three.

1. _____
2. _____
3. _____

Three things I've failed to notice or appreciate about myself are:

1. _____
2. _____
3. _____

Finally, complete the following:

The main reason I'm glad I'm me is:

_____
_____
_____

Congratulations on finding out some of the many wonderful qualities that make you special.

Below is a ten-step action plan to develop cast-iron confidence.

1. Acknowledge you are special and take very good care of yourself. This sends a message to your inner self that you are special and important.
2. Use Reiki to boost your confidence. Give yourself Reiki with the intent that your self-confidence increases every day.
3. Acknowledge your accomplishments. Celebrate your strengths and affirm your successes. Make sure you accept compliments and the credit for your achievements.
4. Appear confident. Even if you aren't feeling it, when you look as if you are, you very often become it. Give yourself Reiki before an important event. Use the absent healing technique learned at Second Degree to send energy in advance to yourself.

5. Don't let setbacks get in the way. Move on after a disappointment. Don't let yourself dwell on things that didn't work out.

6. Honour who you are and expect others to as well. Set high standards in the way you treat yourself and expect no less from the way others treat you.

7. Find the support you need. Get plenty of support and inspiration from a friend or family member or sign up with a life coach. Choose to spend time with friends who make you feel appreciated and understood.

8. Reward yourself. Find ways to reward yourself when you do something that daunted you. By acknowledging your success, you are setting the stage for even greater accomplishment next time.

9. Always take action. It is better to try and learn from your mistakes than never to have had a go at all. Lots of people know what to do, but very few actually do what they know. By taking action, you make the most of every moment. Anthony Robbins says, 'A real decision is measured by the fact that you've taken a new action. If there's no action, you haven't truly decided.'

10. Think positive. To every problem there is always a solution. See every crisis as an opportunity. If you are focused and committed, there is always a way forwards. By sending Reiki to a situation, it is possible to gain greater clarity and move forward with confidence.

Finding your soul mate

It is better to have loved and lost, than never to have loved at all.
ALFRED, LORD TENNYSON

If you feel there is a gap for someone special in your life, Reiki can help you to find the right person. Below is a four-step strategy to help to bring him or her into your life.

I. WHAT DO YOU WANT?

First, it is important for you to think carefully about the type of person you wish to attract. You need to be very specific. What sort of person would make you happy? What character traits would you value, e.g. kindness, generosity, wealth, honesty, etc? What would he or she look like? How tall are they, what age, what colour eyes? What sort of education have they had? What kind of values would such a person have? What sort of job? What kind of lifestyle? Be specific. Don't say rich and then complain when you get a miser. Say financially secure with a generous disposition. Really think of every aspect you can and try to build up a picture of the sort of person you have in mind. Write it all down carefully, sign and date it. Keep it safe.

2. ASK THE UNIVERSE

Tell the universe in detail about the type of person you would like to meet. Ask for help in finding him or her. Explain either out aloud or in your mind exactly what kind of person you are looking for. Know the universe has received your order and trust that everything will work out perfectly.

3. SENT REIKI TO YOUR INTENT

When you receive a Reiki treatment, send the intent that you would like to meet someone special as described on your list. You may want to fold the paper into your hands and send Reiki to the list as well. After this, put the list away and relax.

4. TAKE ACTION

Respond to any instincts you have. Don't just stay at home every evening. Go to places where your future partner is likely to be. Suggestions are:

- Follow your interests and go to places where you are likely to meet up with like-minded people. There are seminars available on just about everything, from self-development to property investment.
- Join an activity group, such as hiking or sailing.
- Make the effort to go to special-interest events, such as concerts, the theatre or art galleries.
- Go to singles events in your area or community.
- If you are not living in the right area to meet the person on your list, move.
- Don't hesitate to use Internet dating sites. If used with common sense, they are an excellent way to meet new people and establish relationships. Make sure you take a few safety precautions, such as not revealing your home address. It is safer to arrange the first meeting in a public place and, of course, never travel in the car of anyone you do not know. Trust your instincts! Visit www.MatchNet.co.uk
- Speed dating is a very enjoyable and effective way of meeting a future partner. There are many organisations on the Internet offering these events. They involve meeting a number of potential partners for just eight minutes each without exchanging any contact details. At the end of the session you write down the names of anyone you would like to see more of. If the other person has written your name down too, then you are each given contact details for the other person. Speed dating can be a lot of fun and is an ideal time to use your intuition to determine whether someone is right for you. Check out www.8minutedating.com

Make the most of every opportunity. Accept unexpected invitations. Listen to your inner voice. If something or someone sounds too good to be true, they will be! Go with your gut instinct. Don't expect movie-style love-at-first-sight meetings. Often instant attraction between two people with seemingly compatible interests or communication styles simply doesn't last. Real love grows over time and involves a conscious choice. It can take a while to develop a relationship and build emotional intimacy. Know that the right person is out there for you and will come into your life at the right time, which is probably when you least expect it. Enjoy the surprises that come your way!

CHAPTER FOURTEEN

Reiki and Terminal Illness

REIKI CAN BE MOST HELPFUL when treating the very ill, the infirm and the terminally ill, as well as benefiting their families and those taking care of them. The carers can always use Reiki to replenish their own energy levels, so that they are more able to provide the support and healing for others. Reiki can be used for pain relief and to provide a nurturing, reassuring connection between the person and those in a caring capacity.

Dr Elisabeth Kubler-Ross pioneered remarkable research with terminally ill patients, ultimately changing for ever our perceptions on this aspect of human experience.

Whilst some religions and sages representing many cultures have always talked of the immortality of the human soul, the subject of death is not something our civilisation is able to discuss easily. Dr Kubler-Ross encouraged patients to speak about their feelings, and discovered that they all shared a tremendous feeling of isolation, as well as fear, and often anger too. With her compassion and warm understanding, Dr Kubler-Ross inspired countless medical staff, care workers and families of terminally ill patients to provide sensitive, responsive care, so that it was possible for each person to die in dignity, surrounded by love.

Princess Diana touched the hearts of millions with her compassion for those who were suffering. Her hospital visits changed the lives of those she visited for ever. She had a rare gift of being able to communicate her empathy with people regardless of their illness or circumstances. She always physically touched those she visited, even if they suffered from a disease considered contagious or dangerous in some way. Whether Princess Diana had ever taken Reiki training is not known, but her instinctive ability to bring comfort to others in pain demonstrates the important element of human touch as used in Reiki.

Many people who have had 'near death experiences' have described remarkably similar journeys towards a bright light. They have nearly all met people whom they either once knew or who were specifically there to accompany them. Yet despite copious amounts of data recording such encounters, many people die alone, in great fear.

Experience with our own parents, as described in the preface of this book, taught us much about the nature of caring for terminally ill people. Since discovering Reiki, we have learned that there is a great difference between healing and curing. Sometimes there simply isn't a cure. Healing can be used and that person may pass away truly at peace with themselves and others, surrounded by their loved ones.

Dr Kubler-Ross defined five stages between the initial reaction of an individual to a diagnosis and the final acceptance of the inevitable. When assisted compassionately throughout, the process becomes considerably easier and can result in that person finding a tremendous amount of peace and harmony that can assist them and all those connected with them to find strength and clarity during a difficult time. She wrote several books on this subject. The following stages are taken from her book *On Death and Dying*.

1. DENIAL AND ISOLATION

Denial is very often the initial reaction of those who are informed as to the terminal nature of their illness. Patients become convinced that there must have been a mistake – 'the X-rays must be mixed up'. Dr Kubler-Ross believes this reaction is one of shock that allows the person time to come to terms with the unexpectedly frightening news. She also suggests it is helpful if the support given during this period allows the individual time to adjust to the diagnosis. Reiki is helpful in treating the shock as well as any symptoms. As mentioned earlier in the book, however, there are times when Reiki is not appropriate (see Chapter Ten).

2. ANGER

The second reaction, after the diagnosis has been accepted, is one of anger and resentment. 'Why me?' 'Why at this time?' This stage is usually more difficult to deal with from the family's viewpoint. Dr Kubler-Ross believes it is important to empathise with the person at this time and be understanding about their predicament. Reiki can be helpful to alleviate any discomfort and reduce the side effects of any treatment that is prescribed.

3. BARGAINING

Following the stage of anger, Dr Kubler-Ross observes that often people will subsequently react by bargaining for more time, such as saying 'If I can just be around for my son's wedding' or 'If only I could be here for the birth of my first grandchild'. Sometimes patients promise that if they can have longer, they will dedicate their lives to God.

Dr Kubler-Ross suggests it would be helpful if these remarks were not just brushed aside by staff, but taken as the beginning of a discussion about any guilt or regret the person may be experiencing at this time in their life.

4. DEPRESSION

Depression is often the next stage, when the person's situation becomes more difficult and they must endure more surgery or more discomfort. There may also be financial burdens that must be faced.

An understanding carer will have no difficulty in establishing the cause of the depression. Reiki may help to deal with the grief that the person is experiencing in order to prepare themselves for the next stage; that of separation from their loved ones.

It is helpful for the person to be assisted in concluding any unfinished business and resolving any conflicts that remain between themselves and their families or other persons close to them. Reiki can often help with any pain relief or to speed up the healing process after surgery has taken place. Additionally it can effectively increase clarity so that the person can become aware of what needs to be done and is able to resolve any remaining difficulties.

5. ACCEPTANCE

If a person has been given enough time and some help in working through the other stages, he or she will become neither angry nor depressed and will reach a stage of acceptance of the inevitable.

This is not necessarily a happier stage. It is a time when the patient will have found some peace and acceptance whilst the rest of the family may themselves be in greater need of help and support.

Often the patient wishes to be left alone at this stage and not to be bothered by the outside world. It may be helpful to visit in silence and show that the person is not alone and is really cared about and supported. Reiki may or may not be refused and the patient could benefit from distant healing at this time. Throughout all these stages hope persists. Even the most accepting patient hopes that a last-minute cure may save them.

When finally there is a time in the patient's life when the pain ceases and the mind drifts off into a dreamless state, it becomes more difficult for the next of kin to know whether to care for the dying or to attend to the needs of the living. Dr Kubler-Ross suggests that the carer could be of great help at this time by selecting the person who feels most comfortable to stay with the dying person. This allows the others to return home without feeling they are abandoning the patient to die alone.

If the person is unconscious, they may still be able to benefit from the Reiki energy, and if they are close to death, they may find they can use the energy to assist them in their transition.

In conclusion, Reiki can provide a gentle and effective means of supporting and helping our loved ones who are seriously or terminally ill. It also allows you to experience a sense of union with the dying person and assists them in coming to terms with their situation.

For what is it to die, but to stand naked in the wind and to melt into the sun?
And what is it to cease breathing, but to free the breath from its restless tides, that it may rise and expand and seek God unencumbered?

Only when you drink from the river of silence shall you indeed sing,
And when you have reached the mountaintop, then you shall begin to climb.
And when the earth shall claim your limbs, then shall you truly dance.

KAHLIL GIBRAN, *THE PROPHET*

Coping with grief

When you part from your friend you grieve not; for that which you love most in him may be clearer in his absence, as the mountain for the climber is clearer from the plain.

KAHLIL GIBRAN, *THE PROPHET*

In religions such as Judaism, Hinduism, Sikhism, Buddhism and Greek Orthodox, there are prescribed ways to deal with loss. Grieving follows a strict formula, usually comprising seven days of deep mourning followed by a gradual decrease over the following twelve months. Such procedures may sound rigid, but they can be surprisingly effective in helping a person, family or group come to terms with losing a loved one. Our secular society has lost this, and people often struggle with repressed emotions and the stiff-upper-lip approach.

There are a number of ways in which you can help. One way is to offer to spend time with bereaved people. There is often no need to talk. Simply being there brings comfort and support. Offer practical help, such as doing shopping or looking after the children. Encourage people to eat and take a multi-vitamin for stability and mental well-being. Make sure they rest, sleep and have some exercise, such as going for a walk or a swim. Offering a Reiki treatment helps too. Homeopathy can also assist, with different remedies prescribed for individual symptoms.

Keeping a grief journal is a powerfully healing and immensely therapeutic tool. People use this journal to record their emotional journey, which helps them through this difficult time. Many people find that attending a support group helps. Others find their pain too difficult to express in front of a group and benefit from grief counselling on a one-to-one basis. Yet others find comfort visiting a church, synagogue, mosque or temple. Everyone reacts differently, and it is important to allow the time and the space to heal the grief. Reiki can help the process by providing comfort and support on a number of levels. It can release trapped emotions that help a person deal with their grief and loss more easily. An organisation called CRUSE offers bereavement counselling. Further information on dealing with grief can be found on their website at www.crusebereavementcare.org.uk (telephone: 0870 167 1677).

CHAPTER FIFTEEN

Reiki for Self-development and Spiritual Growth

*We are not human beings having a spiritual experience. We
are spiritual beings having a human experience.*

TEILHARD DE CHARDIN

Access your inner guidance system

REIKI ENHANCES OUR INNER spiritual connection. We begin to
respond differently, simply becoming more open and loving. Additionally intuition develops and we are able to tap into inner wisdom
and guidance. Personal and spiritual growth is heightened and a multitude of possibilities for accelerating personal growth begin to emerge.
It is possible to learn to sense subtle energies and develop awareness
beyond our five senses, and potentially enter expanded states of
consciousness, where we can discover inner joy, peace and vitality.

Meditation is probably the simplest way to expand consciousness
and tune into your inner guidance. The process of giving or receiving
Reiki enables you to enter a meditative state, often without realising
it. Those who already meditate find their meditations deepen
following Reiki attunements. Reiki and meditation complement
each other.

Meditating for just twenty minutes a day can be an invaluable
way of discovering inner peace and accessing your internal source of
inspiration.

MEDITATION EXERCISE

Sit comfortably upright on a chair, close your eyes and allow yourself to take several slow, deep breaths. Begin to focus all your attention on your breathing, becoming aware of the rhythms as you breathe in and out. Keep your awareness on your breathing without thinking too much about it. Observe its flow. Allow passing thoughts to drift by without becoming involved. If your mind should wander, just gently bring your attention back to your breathing. After about twenty minutes, you may find that your mind becomes still and calm. This will take some practice and you may find you wish to focus your attention on a single word, sound or mantra instead of on your breathing. Sometimes it is necessary to experiment to find what works for you. There is no right or wrong way to meditate. Try to find the method that suits you.

Meditating for about twenty minutes twice a day is ideal. If you are an early riser, sunrise is a good time, especially if busy family life prevents you doing so around breakfast time. Similarly, close to sunset is another time that works well. Both these times herald the change between day and night, which is a special time providing an invaluable space before the day unfolds or the night arrives. When you have been meditating for some time, you can find that you slip into a wonderful space where the mind becomes as still as a forest pool. The nature of reality and ultimate truth begins to unfold and it is possible to find great peace and inner strength.

Visualisation can be helpful as well. Various forms of visualisation are often used on personal development courses and can be employed during Reiki training. In the course of Reiki attunements, participants often experience overwhelming feelings of love and a sense of being connected to all living things. The feeling of love is not of an interpersonal nature; it is more in the realm of universal love.

Whilst Reiki is a route by which to enter expanded states of awareness, visualisation can pave the way to higher levels of mind. Through visualisation, we are able to access that wiser, all-knowing part of ourselves that is often called the higher self, or the soul. Whilst we often struggle with a particular issue, our higher self has a perception of the whole picture and can sense the outcome of a situation. By integrating this expansive aspect of ourselves, we can often access this knowledge and draw inspiration and clarity from a greater perspective.

The following visualisation is a journey to connect with the higher self, in order to experience a higher state of mind. Guided imagery is more effective if you are in a relaxed state of mind. Be open to whatever might happen during this inner journey and trust that it is right for you. You may choose to have someone read this to you as you relax, or record it on to a tape player.

JOURNEY TO THE HIGHER SELF

Imagine you are on a special journey to find your higher self. You are feeling very relaxed as you float gently on in darkness, travelling deeper and deeper into space. As you continue to move deeper into the darkness of inner space, you become aware of a flow of healing warmth that is drawn towards you, and as this flow travels closer to you, it is as if you are being gently enveloped in a gossamer wave of pure love.

It is your higher self, that part from which you were created, the wise, all-knowing centre of your essence, which gently cocoons you in a flow of healing energy, giving you strength and unity, wholeness and harmony. Feel this flow of warmth as it releases all your stresses and strains, allowing energy to flow freely through your system. Let this energy flow through every part of you, at every level. Feel the warmth of the love, as you feel the power of the healing energy flowing through to you from your higher self. Know, too, that the wisdom of the higher self is flowing through to you, filling every part of you, at every level.

As the healing energy flows into your being, allow yourself to relax completely and totally, letting your higher self replenish your system with whatever you need. Feel the wholeness and harmony fill you with peace and tranquillity. When you are ready, slowly and gently return to the room.

An interesting technique for problem-solving is to use internal advisers or inner guides created by the power of our imagination. Such helpers can be Reiki guides, wise sages, figures from history, present-day experts in a particular field or indeed any characters at all, real or fictitious. After a little practice, imaginary conversations can be held and it is possible to gain insight or a wider perspective. It is surprising how helpful this can be. The following meditation is just an example to start the process.

INNER GUIDANCE

Relax deeply and imagine yourself in a beautiful place in nature. Use all your senses to imagine yourself there. Visualise yourself raising your cupped hands in front of you and sending energy streaming out. From this energy, see a stream of light form a white bridge in front of you. Begin walking over the bridge, and as you walk across, allow all tension to disappear and feel yourself filled with relaxation and tranquillity. At the other side of the bridge are some steps leading up a gently sloping hillside. Take the steps to the top, where you will come to a beautiful, shimmering temple surrounded by fragrant, colourful gardens. Standing in the gardens are your advisers, waiting to welcome you. Greet them and spend the next few moments asking for their guidance on any subject at all. You may wish to ask for insight on a particular problem or advice as to the next step in your life's journey, or perhaps about skills and qualities you wish to develop. Listen carefully for the answers. Spend as much time as you wish with your guides, and know that you can return here whenever you need to. When you have finished, gently return down the steps, across the bridge of light and bring yourself back to the room.

OBTAINING ANSWERS TO QUESTIONS

This is another useful technique for receiving answers to questions from your inner guidance resource. Use an alarm clock with a 'snooze' button. When the alarm first rings, pose the question you have in mind to a Reiki guide or another internal adviser, press the snooze button and let yourself fall back to sleep. By the time the alarm rings again, you should have your answer. The early hours are an excellent time to access inner clarification, which is why meditating around sunrise is so appropriate. The mind has usually had time to clear out all the less meaningful thoughts relating to the daily humdrum of our lives, resulting in more significant images and ideas being allowed to surface.

Make time for you

Deep inside all of us is the person we long to be. All too often we define ourselves by the circumstances we find ourselves in, only feeling good about ourselves if things go well. Unless you consciously detach and detoxify yourself emotionally on a regular basis, your self-perception can become heavily clouded by negative, limiting messages received from the world around you. In order to feel clear and wholesome, decide to consciously take time out for the most important person in your life – yourself. Here are some suggestions:

1. Create more time for yourself by delegating some of the jobs others can do for themselves. Instead of focusing on lists and regular obligations, make a not-to-do list, so that you can free yourself up a little. It is a liberating exercise.
2. Find time regularly to be alone, whether outdoors in nature or simply taking an extended bath with your favourite oils and scented candles. You may find time to meditate whilst watching a flickering candle burn, or give yourself a Reiki treatment, sending energy to wash away any accumulated junk messages that don't serve you well.
3. Choose to spend one evening a week doing something you especially enjoy, whether alone or with friends and family. You may choose to have a massage, read a book, take a yoga class, or see a positive, uplifting film with friends. Schedule time for activities you enjoy every week so you don't miss them.

4. Decide to say no or defer making a decision that commits your precious time, energy and focus elsewhere. If you say yes as a matter of course, you'll find yourself regretting and resenting the decision later on. It helps to periodically work out what your values are. This is a powerful way of discovering where your priorities really lie. Then you can become clear about the focus of your life.

5. Choose to manage your time, rather than time managing you, and if all else fails, find fifteen minutes a day for yourself every day, no matter what happens. Make this time sacred, so you can have quality time to yourself and give yourself the nurturing you deserve.

Surround yourself with loving, supportive people

Choose to spend time with people who make you feel positive and enthusiastic about your life and its focus. It's surprising how often we allow ourselves to spend time with those who drain our energy and limit our vision. Anthony Robbins says that it's rare for anyone to rise above the expectations of their peer group. Choose to be an unlimited person and fill your life with those who inspire you and share your positive approach.

Reiki can help you to attract new people. If you would like to bring new relationships into your life, give yourself a Reiki treatment with the intent that you would like to meet more like-minded people. Use visualisation to see yourself socialising with them and enjoying their company. Follow your interests and take time to track down kindred spirits on courses, at clubs or at a support group of some sort. You may choose to make a conscious effort to appreciate the qualities of the friends that you already have. Acknowledging their uniqueness, either verbally or with an appropriate gesture, such as a gift of some sort, can honour them in a very special way and enrich the relationship.

Nurture your spiritual well-being

Spiritual well-being has a different meaning for each one of us. For many, it is about wanting to live more authentically and in tune with our inner wisdom. Everyday life can cause us to lose sight of our spiritual quest, and it can take a conscious effort to re-focus. It can also mean connecting with a higher power on a regular or more frequent basis. Reiki treatments in themselves nurture your spiritual well-being. The following are a few more suggestions to help you honour and align more fully with your own spiritual nature.

TAKE NOTE OF YOUR DREAMS

Dreams have many useful purposes. One is to prepare you for the events you anticipate in the future. The other is to bring about a balance between the opposites that exist within each of us. Dreams and visualisations give us a wealth of resources by providing a valuable pathway into the unconscious mind. If you expect to receive insights in your dreams, it is surprising how often you will. Make a habit of keeping a pen and paper by your bed so that you can make a note of vivid dreams before they fade. Note every element, however insignificant they seem at the time. Record the theme and how you felt during the dream. Even if a dream seems meaningless at the time, it is worth keeping your notes in case they become relevant later on.

MAKE MEDITATION A REGULAR HABIT

By consciously stilling the mind, your inner world is able to communicate with you more easily. Carl Jung believed we are all connected by what he termed the 'collective unconscious', a sort of transpersonal Internet. By allowing ourselves to have regular periods without the sensory input of everyday life, our minds can learn to become detached from everyday concerns. When this happens, it becomes easier to see the nature of things as they really are without being clouded by emotional and other issues. People who regularly meditate find they become more compassionate, understanding and loving.

SOOTHE THE MIND, BODY AND SOUL

Know what nurtures you. Make a conscious effort to listen to your body and get in tune with your physical needs. Rest when you are tired. Chill out when you are stressed. Choose to eat only the finest fresh produce, and exercise on a regular basis to keep yourself balanced and healthy.

Seek out healthy verbal environments. Words impact on every cell in your body and each response affects you at every level. Make a determined effort to surround yourself with people whose company you enjoy and whose attitude and words uplift you.

Make your home a place you look forward to returning to. Create a serene and harmonious environment that provides a sanctuary from a stress-filled world. Decorate with harmonious colours that are easy to live with, and include different ways to nourish the senses and soothe the soul.

BE KIND TO OTHERS

Gestures of kindness (especially unexpected ones) are great sources of joy both for the receiver and also for the giver. Take time to notice what makes others happy and, if you can, do something for them, especially something they wouldn't do for themselves.

Kahlil Gibran, the poet, eloquently expresses the joy of giving in his book *The Prophet*, from which the following is taken:

There are those who give little of the much they have – and they give it for recognition, and their hidden desire makes their gift unwholesome.

And there are those who have little to give and give it all.
These are the believers in life and the bounty of life and their
coffers are never empty.

Working with others to help those in need is a wonderful way to combine resources and improve the lives of those in your community. If you suspect that someone could use a hand, you are probably right. However, kindness should be offered in a thoughtful and appropriate way. We cannot assume we know the needs of others. Sometimes empathy is all that is needed; at other times it may be practical help or motivation to change their circumstances. Kindness to others honours and nurtures them. In giving, you are enriched. Many people, including life coach Anthony Robbins, believe that serving others is the secret to happiness and fulfilment.

KEEP A JOURNAL

A journal can bring a special dimension to your life by capturing insights and experiences that would otherwise be forgotten. When imaginatively used, journal writing can also be a helpful way of exploring ideas, feelings and spiritual desires. It is a place where coincidences and synchronicities can be noted. Inspirational quotations can be stored, spiritual experiences can be recorded. Sometimes, when words are not enough, use drawings to express your feelings more adequately. Drawing and painting is a useful and therapeutic way of accessing the subconscious mind. A journal can also be used to keep the answers to self-development exercises completed on courses or in books or magazines. Journal writing can provide a sacred space during a busy day and a fascinating record of desires and insights to look back upon later.

GIVE AND RECEIVE REIKI TREATMENTS

A Reiki treatment is a wonderful way to nurture yourself, and enhance your physical, mental, emotional and spiritual well-being. If you already practise Reiki, find like-minded others you can spend time with, so that you can give and receive treatments on a regular basis.

CHAPTER SIXTEEN

Becoming a Reiki Practitioner

THE ONLY NECESSARY REQUIREMENT for becoming a Reiki practitioner is to have an open heart, the desire to receive the attunements and the intention to use Reiki to heal and help others. Reiki has grown considerably in popularity over the past ten years, and there is much demand for practitioners. It will probably be helpful, if you intend to practise Reiki on a professional basis, to join either a complementary therapy organisation or a Reiki practitioners' association. They will provide valuable contacts with other practitioners and keep you informed of any new developments. A list of such organisations is at the back of the book.

Before opening your door to clients, it is important to find out if there are any specific laws pertaining to non-medical practitioners where you live, just in case there are regulations you need to be aware of. Your Reiki Master should be able to advise you on this.

INSURANCE

Whereas the Usui System of Reiki in itself is not harmful, and only serves to break down the barriers to harmony, it is as well to have insurance if you are a professional practitioner of any persuasion. Personal indemnity insurance is essential. If you are already practising another healing art, it may be possible to add Reiki to the policy.

Most insurance companies can provide a quotation for this, and in many countries there are specialist insurance companies who provide policies especially for those working in the caring professions. It is also recommended that you take out liability insurance to protect yourself from litigation should a person sustain accidental damage to themselves, such as falling down the stairs at your home or slipping over whilst getting off the treatment table. If you work at a clinic, they will probably have this insurance already.

EXPERIENCE

If you do not feel confident enough, practise more on your family and friends. Take your time. If there is no one you can practise with, find out where your local sharing group is held and join other Reiki people there.

If you haven't used Reiki for a long time, ask your Reiki Master if you can sit in again on First Degree and refresh yourself. You may wish to spend some time offering Reiki to people in hospitals or hospices. Often maternity units welcome healers to treat expectant mothers.

If your aim is to get more experience, offer to help giving treatments at Reiki stands at exhibitions in your area. You may decide to get together with other practitioners and take a stand yourself. It is surprising how much people benefit from treatment at these events despite the noisy environment.

CLIENT RECORDS

It is also recommended that you keep client records for some time, to ensure that details are available should they be required in the future, for any reason, however unlikely. These need not be extensive and should ideally include the name, address and telephone number of the person, together with their doctor's address and contact number. Additionally it would be wise to record any medication they may be taking and if they have any artificial aids such as a pacemaker fitted. It is of course never appropriate to ask clients to alter the medication they have been prescribed by their doctor. It would be useful to record the reason for their treatment and whether they have been treated for any mental or physical disorders. Note any allergies or phobias they suffer from.

CONFIDENTIALITY

Confidentiality is an important part of any professional relationship. If you feel there are certain circumstances where you could not guarantee to maintain confidentiality, for example, if you think they might harm themselves or others, then this must be mentioned at an early stage.

WHEN REIKI IS NOT APPROPRIATE

It is sensible to be aware of when Reiki is not an appropriate treatment. This is covered fully in Chapter Ten.

ADVERTISING

Many of your clients will come to you because they have been personally recommended to do so, which is the best way. To let people know what you do, it is helpful to have some small brochures printed explaining what Reiki is and where you can be contacted. When you have gained sufficient experience and confidence, you may wish to let local holistic centres know that you are a Reiki practitioner and could offer their clients treatments on certain days of the week or when required.

Should you decide to have cards printed with your details, it is advisable not to include your home address. Print your details and telephone number only. Post details locally at places with community notice boards. Ask your local library, gym and health food shop whether you can display your cards. Hand them out wherever you go to let people know what you are offering. Practitioners' associations will often publicise your details on their websites. Find out if the Master you trained with has a website and see if your details can be included.

TREATMENT COUCH

Your local clinic or healing centre may have treatment tables you can use, or you may decide to invest in one for your own use. There are many options available and it is well to remember that most are designed for massage and are understandably sturdy. It is not necessary to buy such a table for Reiki unless you practise some form of holistic massage as well. Nor would a table need to be exceptionally wide. Your own comfort is paramount when giving a treatment, and you would not wish to be stretching across an unnecessarily large area. It is advisable to find a table that is strong and as light as possible but which is the right height for you to work on without straining your own back.

Many of these tables flatteringly named 'portable' are probably better described as 'luggable'. It is preferable to buy one that you can easily manoeuvre, rather than one that requires a couple of weight-lifters to transport for you. If you can find a table which allows you to pull up a chair at the head and possibly the foot, you may well find this a useful feature. When treating the head positions especially, it is helpful to have the option of being seated, resting the elbows comfortably on the table either side of the person's head. At the Reiki School, we have tables built especially for us – details on page 164.

CHARGES FOR TREATMENT

If you are only treating your family, there will be no need to charge, as it is all good practice. Once you decide to become a professional practitioner, you will need to have a scale of charges for the treatments you give to cover your costs and pay your own bills.

If you are in a situation where you are helping on a voluntary basis, then it may not be appropriate to charge for your time. If you are paying for the use of a room in a holistic centre and incurring costs advertising your treatment, then it would be sensible to make a charge for your work.

Many practitioners offer a discount, if a course of several treatments is booked in advance. It is a sad fact of human nature that people do not appreciate what they receive free of charge. Many practitioners who do not charge are often less busy and are frequently let down at the last minute, whereas those charging a high price are booked for months in advance and have a waiting list. Some people simply don't feel comfortable having an obligation to others that they are unlikely to be able to repay.

You may, however, feel you would like to offer treatment at a concessionary rate to disadvantaged persons, such as those who are unemployed or disabled.

COPING WITH EMOTIONS

In a loving, caring environment, it is not unusual to find that clients are able to bring up deep-seated emotions and difficult past experiences. It is helpful to keep a box of paper tissues in your therapy room for this purpose. Expressing grief, sadness, anger, fear or whatever emotion has been buried helps to heal pain.

Our culture often encourages us to 'be brave' and 'soldier on' when we would rather allow ourselves to feel vulnerable and acknowledge our feelings. The gradual growth process that accompanies Reiki training often provides a safe space for us to face and deal with emotional issues. Only from personal experience and growth in this area can a practitioner provide the empathy, understanding and support to another, who is facing a difficult time emotionally, brought to the surface by the Reiki treatment.

Providing a safe, loving, supportive environment allows people to shed their tears and release their sadness. Often this outpouring of emotion will herald a turning point in their healing process.

SOME PRACTICAL DETAILS FOR GIVING A REIKI TREATMENT

Expect to spend a few minutes talking to your client before a treatment. Ask why they have come, and what symptoms they are experiencing. Ask briefly and non-intrusively about their family background and present circumstances. Explain what to expect from a treatment.

- Wash your hands before and after treatment.
- Be sure to remove watches and rings.
- Make sure your breath is fresh – don't eat spicy food before a treatment.
- Breathe away from the person.
- Use tranquil, meditative music to accompany treatments.
- Use the positions as a guide, but act intuitively when placing hands.
- Wear clean, comfortable, lightweight clothing, preferably in layers, so that you do not become overheated. We don't recommend anyone offer treatments in a medical-style white coat.
- Place the hands on the body without undue pressure.
- Keep the hands away from the nose and throat and other sensitive areas.
- Try to keep contact with the body or the auric field in between positions, as appropriate.
- Warn the recipient they may experience detoxification symptoms.
- Be as relaxed as you can.
- Allow some time after the treatment for the client to rest and regain their composure.
- Allow yourself a few minutes in between treatments.

In Conclusion

The best and most beautiful things in the world cannot be seen, nor touched . . . but are felt in the heart.

HELEN KELLER

IN THIS BOOK, WE HAVE attempted to clarify a healing art that is simple and enigmatic, straightforward yet mysterious. Reiki brings about a subtle inner shift that forever changes the perception of those drawn to it, opening their hearts and minds to infinite possibilities. It is intangible, yet can be perceived by the senses. With it, each person can move closer to a state of wholeness and balance.

Overall, Reiki is a powerful tool for raising self-awareness and enabling us to participate in our own healing process. By leading us to the cause of our own suffering, we are better able to assist others to do likewise.

It can help to uncover aspects of ourselves that we were previously unaware of. Through the discovery of our own qualities and abilities, we are then able to embrace others with more compassion and understanding.

When we reach a turning point in our own lives, the clarity and the increased awareness can help us to determine the next step. Reiki enables us to respond with love instead of fear and move forward with confidence instead of uncertainty. Our vision of how our life can be will create that life. Seeing through present obstacles will take us beyond them and give us the confidence to trust that things will always work out for the best in the end.

The healing energy of Reiki could be said to equate to love. Pure, unconditional love transcends all barriers and restores equilibrium within the body, mind and spirit, bringing joy in its wake.

Life is a song – sing it
Life is a game – play it
Life is a challenge – meet it
Life is a dream – realise it
Life is a sacrifice – offer it
Life is love – enjoy it

Sai Baba

The Reiki School

If you have any questions, comments or stories to share, please write in or send a text message or an email. Whilst we welcome your feedback and will reply to all letters and emails, this may take some time due to our travel commitments. We can be contacted at:

The Reiki School
Budworth
Shay Lane
Hale
Altrincham
WA15 8UE
UK
Tel/Fax: 0161 980 6453
Mobile: 07968 352 952
Email: info@thereikischool.co.uk
Website: www.thereikischool.co.uk

Treatment tables and specially adapted CDs for Reiki treatments are available direct from the Reiki School. Courses are held in many parts of the UK and overseas. A current schedule of events is available on the website above or can be obtained by email or telephone request.

Useful Websites

REIKI ASSOCIATIONS AND OTHER CENTRES

The Reiki Association (UK)
www.reikiassociation.org

The Reiki Alliance
www.reikialliance.com

UK Reiki Federation
www.reikifed.co.uk

International Association of Reiki Professionals (USA)
www.iarp.org

The Australian Reiki Connection (Aus)
www.australianreikiconnection.com.au

Canadian Reiki Association
www.reiki.ca

The Reiki Association of South Africa
www.reikiassociation.co.za

Reiki New Zealand Inc.
www.reiki.org.nz

Reiki Outreach
www.annieo.com/reikioutreach

The Reiki School & Clinic (USA)
www.thereikischool.com

International Institute of Reiki Training (Aus)
www.taoofreiki.com

HEALTH PRACTITIONER ORGANISATIONS

British Complementary Medical Association
www.bcma.co.uk

Complementary Medical Association
www.the-cma.org.uk

International Guild of Professional Practitioners
www.igpp.co.uk

INSURANCE

Independent Professional Therapists International (Insurance)
www.iptiuk.com

H. & L. Balen & Co (Insurance for health practitioners)
www.balen.co.uk

OTHER USEFUL WEBSITES

Eat Right For Your Type
www.dadamo.com

Novo by Immogenics
www.immogenics.com

Susanne Sawyer, Nutritional Therapist and Immunogenic Practitioner
Tel: 01273 834246

Leslie Kenton's books on health and beauty, including information on Syndrome X
www.lesliekenton.com

Stephen Haynes Clairvoyant Life Guide
www.selfpower.com

Violent Hill Studios (Centre for Healing Arts, London)
www.violethillstudios.com

Further Reading

Brennan, Barbara Ann, *Light Emerging*, Bantam, 1994

Brennan, Barbara, *Hands of Light*, New York, Bantam, 1988

Brown, Fran, *Living Reiki – Takata's Teachings*, Life Rhythm, 1992

Coelho, Paolo, *The Alchemist*, HarperCollins, London, 1993

Cohen, Pete, *Habit Busting: A Ten Step Plan That Will Change Your Life*, HarperCollins, 2002

D'Adamo, Peter, *Eat Right For Your Type*, Century Books, 2001

Dethlefsen, T., and Dahlke, R., *The Healing Power of Illness*, Vegas, Shaftesbury, 2002

Edwards, Gill, *Living Magically*, Piatkus, 1999

Ellyard, L., *Reiki Healer*, Lotus Press, 2004

Ellyard, L., *Reiki Satsang*, Healing Traditions Press, 2004

Field, Lynda, *Weekend Life Coach: How to get the life you want in 48 Hours*, Vermilion, 2004

Fontana, David, *The Language of Symbols*, Duncan Baird, 2003

Forster, Mark, *Get Everything Done and Still Have Time to Play*, Hodder & Stoughton, 2000

George, Mike, *1001 Ways to Relax*, Duncan Baird, 2003

Gibran, Kahlil, *The Prophet*, Penguin Books, 2004

Gray, John, *Mars and Venus Starting Over*, Vermilion, 1998

Greaves, Suzy, *Making the Big Leap*, New Holland, 2004

Haberly, Helen, *Reiki – Hawayo Takata's Story*, Archdigm Publications, 2000

Hall, Mari, *Practical Reiki – A Practical Step by Step Guide to Healing*, Thorsons, 1997

Hall, Mari, *Reiki for Common Ailments*, Piatkus, 1999

Hall, Mari, *Reiki for the Soul*, Thorsons, 2000

Harrold, Fiona, *Seven Steps to a New You*, Piatkus, 2004

Hay, Louise, *Heal Your Body*, Hay House, 2004

Hay, Louise, *You Can Heal Your Life*, Hay House, 2002

Haynes, Alison, *Change: How to Kickstart the Future and Refresh the Spirit*, Murdoch, 2004

HH Dalai Lama, *The Art of Happiness*, Hodder & Stoughton, 1999

Holford, Patrick, *The Optimum Nutrition Bible*, Piatkus, 1998

Honervogt, Tanmaya, *Reiki*, Gaia, 1998

Horan, Paula, *Abundance through Reiki*, Lotus Press, 1996

Horan, Paula, *Empowerment Through Reiki*, USA, Lotus Press, 1995

Horan, Paula, *Reiki: 108 Questions & Answers*, Full Circle, 2003

Horan, Paula, *The Ultimate Reiki Touch*, Full Circle Publishing, 1999

Jeffers, Susan, *The Little Book of Confidence*, Vermilion, 1999

Katie, Byron, *Loving What Is*, Ebury Press, 2002

Kenton, Leslie, *The New Raw Energy*, Vermilion, 2001

Kenton, Leslie, *The Powerhouse Diet*, Vermilion, 2004

Kenton, Leslie, *The X-Factor Diet*, Vermilion, 2005

Kingston, Karen, *Clear Your Clutter with Feng Shui*, Piatkus, 1998

Kingston, Karen, *Clutter Free in 7 Days*, Piatkus, 2003

Kubler-Ross, Elisabeth, *Living with Death and Dying*, Souvenir Press, 1998

Kubler-Ross, Elisabeth, *On Death and Dying*, Simon & Schuster, 1987

Lubeck, W., Petter, F., Rand, W., *The Spirit of Reiki*, Lotus Press, 2001

Lubeck, Walter, *The Aura Healing Handbook*, Lotus Press, 2000

Lubeck, Walter, *Reiki Best Practices*, Lotus Press, 2003

Matthews, Andrew, *Follow Your Heart: Finding Purpose in your life and work*, Seashell Books, 1997

McKenna, Paul, *Change Your Life in Seven Days*, Transworld Publishers, 2003

McMillen, Kim, *When I Loved Myself Enough*, Pan McMillan, 2001

Nolen-Hoeksema, Susan, *Women Who Think Too Much*, Piatkus, 2004

Parkes, Chris and Penny, *15-Minute Reiki*, Thorsons, 2004

Quest, Penelope, *Reiki for Life*, Piatkus, 2002

Richardson, Pam, *The Life Coach: Be the person you've always wanted to be*, Hamlyn, 2004

Robbins, Anthony, *Awaken the Giant Within*, Pocket Books, 2004

Robbins, Anthony, *Unlimited Power*, Pocket Books, 2001

Rogers, Rita, *Learning to Live Again: A Practical Spiritual Guide to Coping with Bereavement*, Pan McMillan, 2003

Schinn, Florence Scovel, *The Game of Life and How to Play It*, Vermilion, 2005

Stiene, Bronwen and Frans, *The Reiki Sourcebook*, O Books, 2003

Walsch, Neale Donald, *Conversations with God 1, 2 & 3*, Hodder Mobius, 1997, 1999

Walsch, Neale Donald, *Tomorrow's God*, Hodder & Stoughton, 2004

Walter, Dawna, *How to Do Absolutely Everything*, Quadrille Publishing, 2004

Weil, Andrew, *Eating Well for Optimum Health*, Time Warner, 2000

Weil, Andrew, *8 Weeks to Optimum Health*, Time Warner, 1998

Weil, Andrew, *Spontaneous Healing*, Random House, 1995

Wilde, Stuart, *Infinite Self*, Hay House Inc., 1996

Wilde, Stuart, *The Trick to Money is Having Some*, Hay House, 1995

Index